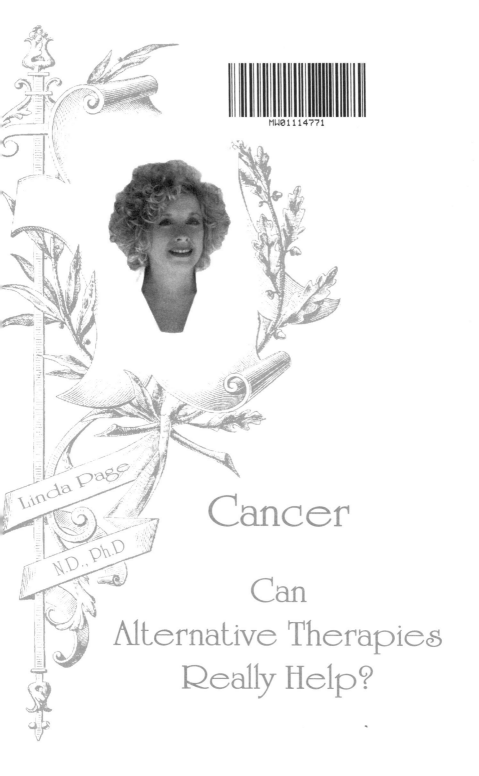

Linda Page

N.D., Ph.D

Cancer

Can
Alternative Therapies
Really Help?

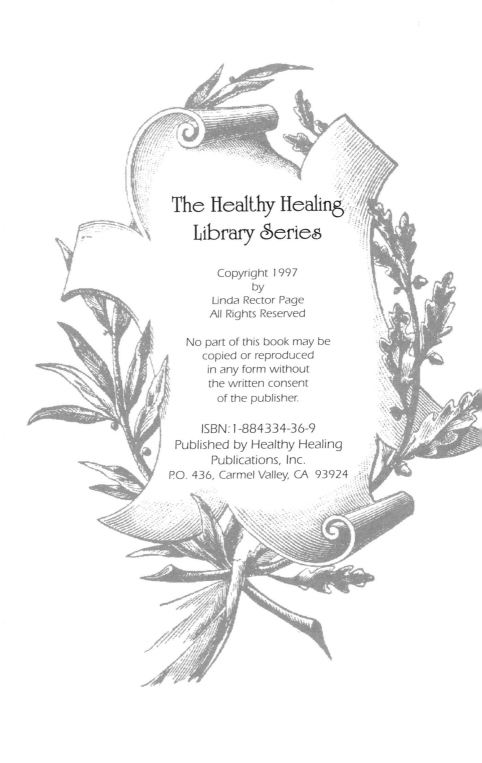

The Healthy Healing Library Series

Copyright 1997
by
Linda Rector Page
All Rights Reserved

No part of this book may be
copied or reproduced
in any form without
the written consent
of the publisher.

ISBN:1-884334-36-9
Published by Healthy Healing
Publications, Inc.
P.O. 436, Carmel Valley, CA 93924

About the Author....

L inda Page has been working in the fields of nutrition and herbal medicine both professionally and as a personal lifestyle choice, since the early seventies. She is a certified Doctor of Naturopathy and Ph.D., with extensive experience in formulating herbal combinations. She received a Doctorate of Naturopathy from the Clayton College of Natural Health in 1988, and a Ph.D. in Nutritional Therapy from the American Holistic College of Nutrition in 1989. She is a member of both the American and California Naturopathic Medical Associations.

Linda opened and operated the "Rainbow Kitchen," a natural foods restaurant, then became a working partner in The Country Store Natural Foods store. Linda is also the founder and formulator of Crystal Star Herbal Nutrition, a manufacturer of over 250 premier herbal compounds. A major, cutting edge influence in the herbal medicine field, Crystal Star Herbal Nutrition products are carried by over twenty-five hundred natural food stores in the U.S. and around the world.

Linda has written four successful books and a Library Series of specialty books in the field of natural healing. Today, she is the editor-in-chief of a national monthly, natural health newsletter, The Natural Healing Report. She has a weekly CBS News TV segment where she discusses a wide range of natural healing topics, and she has her own weekly, one-hour radio talk show program called "The World of Healthy Healing." Linda also lectures around the country, contributes articles to national publications, is regularly featured on radio and television, and is an adjunct professor at Clayton College of Natural Health.

Continuous research in all aspects of the alternative healing world has been the cornerstone of success for her reference work Healthy Healing now in its tenth edition, with sales of almost a million books.

Cooking For Healthy Healing, now in its second revised edition, is a companion to Healthy Healing. It draws on both the recipes from the Rainbow Kitchen and the more defined, lifestyle diets that she has developed for healing. This book contains thirty-three diet programs, and over 900 healthy recipes.

In How To be Your Own Herbal Pharmacist, Linda addresses the rising appeal of herbs and herbal healing in America. This book is designed for those wishing to take more definitive responsibility for their health through individually developed herbal combinations.

Another popular work is Linda's party reference book, Party Lights, written with restaurateur and chef Doug Vanderberg. Party Lights, takes healthy cooking one step further by adding fun to a good diet.

Published by Healthy Healing Publications, 1997

Bibliography & Other Reading

Quillin, Patrick, PhD, R.D., *Beating Cancer with Nutrition.* 1994

Thomas, Richard. *The Essiac Report - Canada's Remarkable Unknown Cancer Remedy.* 1993

Chichoke, Anthony J. *Enzymes & Enzyme Therapy.* 1994

Whitaker, Julian, M.D. The Prostate Report. 1997

Gates, Donna. *The Body Ecology Diet.* 1996

Hershoff, Asa, D.C., N.D. *Homeopathy for Musculoskeletal Healing.* 1996

Stine, Jerry. "Lactoferrin: First Food for Life." *NutriCology - In Focus.* 1997

Mead, Nathaniel, "Reversing Cancer Through Building Immune Health." *Alternative Medicine Digest.* Issue 12

"Modified Citrus Pectin Inhibits Cancer Metastasis." *Life Extension.* Sept. 1996

"Life Extension Research." *Life Extension.* Oct.1997

"Broccoli - Cancer-Fighting Agents." *Better Nutrition for Today's Living.* 1994

"Research News - Smoking Linked to Colo-Rectal Cancer." *Whole Foods.* Ap.1994

Snow, Joanne. "Green Tea Monograph." *Herbclip.* June 1997

Mayne, Susan Taylor, Ph. D., et al. "Dietary Beta Carotene and Lung Cancer Risk in U.S. Non-Smokers." *Journal of the National Cancer Institute.* Jan. 1994

"Green Tea and the Risk of Gastrointestinal Cancers." *Quarterly Review of Natural Medicine.* Summer 1997

"Green Tea Inhibits Experimentally Induced Lung Carcinoma." *Quarterly Review of Natural Medicine.* 1996

Quarterly Review of Natural Medicine. Summer, 1995

Duke, James A., Ph. D. *The Green Pharmacy.* 1997

Books In
The Library
Series

Dr. Page's written papers are thoroughly researched - through empirical observation as well as from documented evidence. Studies are ongoing and updated at Healthy Healing Publications, P.O. Box 436, Carmel Valley, CA 93924

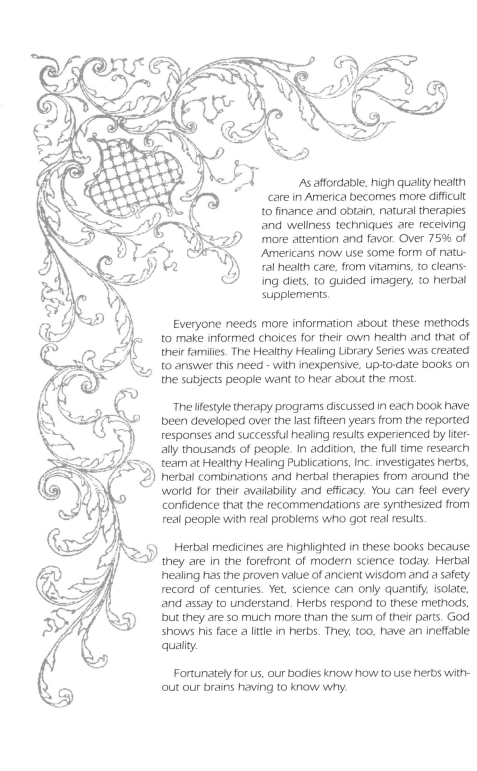

As affordable, high quality health care in America becomes more difficult to finance and obtain, natural therapies and wellness techniques are receiving more attention and favor. Over 75% of Americans now use some form of natural health care, from vitamins, to cleansing diets, to guided imagery, to herbal supplements.

Everyone needs more information about these methods to make informed choices for their own health and that of their families. The Healthy Healing Library Series was created to answer this need - with inexpensive, up-to-date books on the subjects people want to hear about the most.

The lifestyle therapy programs discussed in each book have been developed over the last fifteen years from the reported responses and successful healing results experienced by literally thousands of people. In addition, the full time research team at Healthy Healing Publications, Inc. investigates herbs, herbal combinations and herbal therapies from around the world for their availability and efficacy. You can feel every confidence that the recommendations are synthesized from real people with real problems who got real results.

Herbal medicines are highlighted in these books because they are in the forefront of modern science today. Herbal healing has the proven value of ancient wisdom and a safety record of centuries. Yet, science can only quantify, isolate, and assay to understand. Herbs respond to these methods, but they are so much more than the sum of their parts. God shows his face a little in herbs. They, too, have an ineffable quality.

Fortunately for us, our bodies know how to use herbs without our brains having to know why.

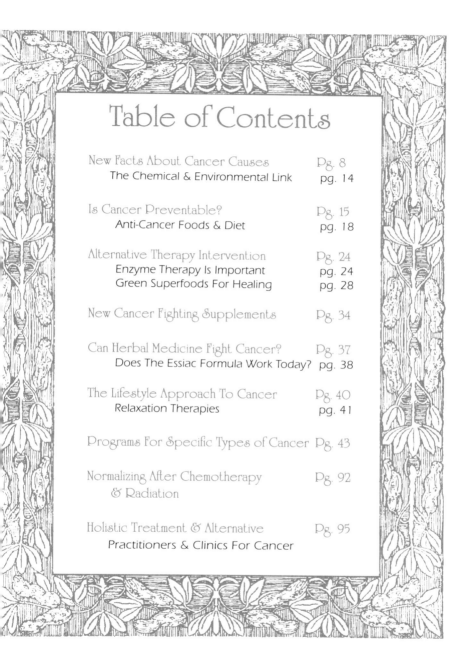

Table of Contents

New Facts About Cancer Causes

Cancer may be reaching epidemic proportions. By the turn of the century, cancer is expected to be the number one cause of death in America. Cancer used to be extremely rare. Is our late twentieth century lifestyle really that bad?

Cancer used to be an uncommon disease. Its dramatic, late 20th century increase is only minimally due to new diagnostic tests like better mammograms, or to calling old diseases like consumption, cancers. The devastating disease we know as cancer today actually emerged gradually and then started rising at extraordinary rates as industrial societies became more and more dependent on technology instead of nature.

What's the report card for our National War On Cancer?

It has been more than twenty-seven years since America officially declared its highly publicized war on cancer. Six and a half million people, *enough for a holocaust*, have died from cancer during those years. American science now has several decades of state-of-the-art research into cancer. We have spent over one trillion dollars in the research effort against this degenerative disease. Yet the report card looks bleak. It seems we are no closer to a "cancer answer" than ever. In fact, the newest statistics show a worsening situation.

1) In 1900, cancer was the sixth or seventh cause of death in America. By 1971, the chances of falling victim to cancer were one in six. By 1983 those chances doubled to one in three. Today, **more than one in three Americans will get cancer.** One in four of those will die from it.

2) **One and a quarter million** Americans will be diagnosed with cancer this year alone! At any given moment, **two and a half million** people are being treated for cancers. Almost half a million Americans die of cancer every year.

3) **Cancer kills more Americans each year than ten times the total of all AIDS fatalities** since the discovery of the HIV virus.

4) Cancer is expected to overtake heart disease as the number one cause of death in America by the year 2000.

While admitting that even though well funded, research successes have been lacking or inconclusive, the National Cancer Institute says that there are bright spots.

Testicular cancer, Hodgkin's disease and childhood leukemia have become treatable. Women diagnosed with breast cancer may now choose a breast-sparing lumpectomy and radiation, instead of a radical mastectomy. Improvements in the surgical technique for colon cancer, a disease that almost always required a colostomy in times past, now allow most patients to keep significant amounts of colon structure.

Cryotherapy, a form of cancer tumor eradication that is less insulting to the body than conventional surgery, shows much promise, even though it cannot help all kinds of cancers, and has many caveats attached to its use.

A new five-year study shows survival rates of cancer patients have increased from 20% of cancer patients in 1930, to 38% in 1971, to 53% of adults and 70% of children today. Most experts, however, feel the NCI data is flawed since it does not include non-whites, and the greatest incidence of new cancers is appearing in blacks, urban poor and workers exposed to toxic substances. Yet, even the current debatable data from the National Cancer Institute shows that less than 10% of victims with cancers of the pancreas, liver, stomach, brain or esophagus will be alive in five years. Many experts assign the blame for the disheartening statistics to the aging of America's population. But, this hardly explains the 28% rise in childhood cancers from 1950 to 1987, or the almost 45% rise during the decade between 1985 and 1995.

In fact, the newest studies, which detail types of cancer by areas of the country, are frightening indeed. Most of these studies show that people who live in high agricultural sections of the U.S. have a dramatically increased risk for hormone-driven cancers, like breast, prostate, endometrial and ovarian cancers. Especially in California, the correlation between these types of cancers and the pounds of organochlorine pesticides used in the foremost growing areas is undeniable. One radio show in January 1997 reported that Northern California had 12 new cases, and 3 deaths from cancer every single day! The same sad statistics are surfacing from Florida, Texas and the Midwest as well.

Why hasn't science made more progress? One of the main problems is the enormous cost of all areas of cancer treatment - from the newest imaging and radiation equipment, to FDA regulations, to insurance payments. It seems unbelievable, but there are still only the same three weapons in the "approved" cancer fighting arsenal - chemotherapy, radiation and surgery. In fact, the vast majority of the funds provided by the National Cancer Act support research to improve the effectiveness of these three existing therapies that have been available for decades. So patients are still being treated with the same three therapies, just more precisely. Chemotherapy is now less toxic, and new medications reduce the nausea and vomiting once considered unavoidable side effects.

One of the main stumbling blocks is that it is proving almost impossible to kill all cancer cells without damaging healthy cells. Chemotherapy and radiation kill malignant cells, harm non-cancerous cells and severely reduce the immune systems' ability to fight off disease. If even one cell is resistant, it will survive and grow into a new tumor. Worse, the new cancer will be impervious to chemotherapy treatment. Of the 500,000 people who die each year of cancer, only 2 to 3% of them benefit from chemotherapy. Radiation treated patients have

severe, long-lasting side effects, like ulcers, painful sores, reproductive malfunction and chronic diarrhea. Many even develop
other cancers because the risk for leukemia is so greatly increased. The traditional medical community today realizes the
downsides and limits to these treatments, admitting that non-
traditional, innovative means must be developed for long-lasting success against cancer.

**Has science made *any* progress, since both the inci-
dence of cancer and death rates continue to climb?**

Most scientists admit that current treatments have been
pushed to their limits. They believe the only hope for the 50%
of patients who can't be helped by conventional therapies lies
in laboratories, where molecular biologists have spent the past
25 years trying to pry the lid off the "black-box" of the cancer
cell. Molecular research has convinced most scientists that cancer is a result of DNA "gone bad." in which inherited or ac-
quired mutations damage the genes that control cell division.

DNA is the master molecule that encodes the genetic script
for every individual life. Amazingly complex, DNA code contains more than 3 billion characters which it replicates as cells
divide. Scientists estimate that **each** of our 60 trillion body cells
undergoes from 1,000 to 10,000 potential cancer-causing DNA
breaks every day. Yet, our DNA repair mechanisms and immune defenses keep genetic damage under control 99% of
the time.

Occasionally, however, there are mistakes during replica-
tion. Cells with DNA defects that are not repaired continue to
divide, and eventually form small abnormal cell growths. The
growths are not always cancerous, but the more cell division
cycles the body undergoes, the more likely it is to accumulate
abnormal cell colonies. This is one of the reasons we are more
likely to see cancer or pre-cancerous conditions after middle
age.

Though cancerous cells divide more rapidly than healthy cells, most cancers take years to form. Cancer caused by defective DNA may take 5 years to develop a tumor 1mm in diameter. Even if it is malignant at this stage, it is not considered dangerous, because the growth's center cells are too far from the bloodstream nutrient supply. And, though new defective cells may be forming, the growth loses old ones just like the rest of the body, so that years and even decades may pass without significant problems.

The real trouble begins when the cancerous cells begin secreting chemicals that attract endothelial cells - the key components of blood vessels. The endothelial cells form capillaries which grow into the tumor and provide the tumor cells with nourishment. They also pump out molecular messengers called Growth Factors that stimulate the tumor to divide more rapidly.

This activity is called **angiogenesis,** a process of blood vessel formation that normally only occurs in growing children. In adults, angiogenesis is seen only during pregnancy, wound healing or certain heart conditions. Angiogenesis around malignant cancer cells creates a nourishment route for the cells to break away from the main tumor mass and migrate to other parts of the body, where they start new malignant colonies. This is the dangerous process called metastasis, and is really the cause of death from cancer. Very few cancer victims die of the primary tumor mass, but rather from the smothering of the body's normal processes due to metastasis.

Can we prevent DNA damage in the first place? DNA damagers can be viruses, radiation, environmental toxins, defective inherited genes, or a combination of these things. Harmful genetic mutations can also result from a diet with excess fat (because fat is involved in hormone activity), or from exposure to carcinogenic chemicals.

Cancer science today revolves around trying to identify the specific genes where damage occurs, and, it is hoped, in finding a way to fix them. This hope largely consists, at present, of using technology that enables biologists to redesign cells from selected pieces of genetic material to create a genetic arsenal that will work against cancer cells - especially cells that produce natural anti-cancer chemicals, or contain cancer-killing properties that nature doesn't provide. Interleukin-2, which intensifies the immune attack response on cancer cells, and tumor necrosis factor (TNF), which disrupts a tumor's blood supply, are two of the most promising.

Yet, while being respectful of all ways of healing, we should also be quite careful about the long range consequences of genetic engineering. The drug world is already crowded with drugs that increase the risk of cancer, drugs that work at far less elemental body levels than our genes.

Heroic medicine such as this tends to hit the body over the head with a chemical hammer, does not address the cause of the problem, and in my opinion, can never take into account all of the complexities and ramifications of "playing God" through genetic construction.

Jurassic Park may only be the first terrifying forerunner of science trying hopelessly to control and predict Nature, which is fundamentally illogical, uncontrollable and unpredictable.

Let's take a look at some of the factors that cause cancer. Although hereditary factors have gotten the media attention lately, in truth, few gene mutations are hereditary. Environmental factors are far more significant in cancer occurrence.

Environmental pollutants are putting large segments of the population at risk by reducing immune functions. Clinical studies show that environmental toxins can damage cell DNA, which leads to cell mutation and tumor development.

Recent World Health Organization studies show that chemical and environmental factors are responsible for 80 to 90% of all cancers. These factors also affect immune response, so the body, instead of defending us, sometimes attacks healthy cells as well, aggravating abnormal growth.

Of the 5 million registered chemicals in the world, people come in contact with 70,000 of them regularly, and at least 20,000 are known carcinogens. **The latest figures show that 25,000 new chemicals enter our culture each year, many of them carried on the winds from third world countries that have few safeguards in place.** U.S. industries alone generate **88 billion pounds** of toxic waste per year. The EPA estimates 90% of them are improperly disposed of. These are frightening numbers indeed!

Many substances that have long been banned in the U.S. continue to present dangers. Two examples are DDT and PCBs, the organo-chlorides used in insecticides and electrical components. The U.S. banned them in the 1970's, but residues still persist in our soil and water. We also sold these chemicals to Third World countries, so sprayed produce from their agriculture continues to come back to us. Although regulatory agencies monitor environmental chemicals, thousands of new ones are constantly entering our air and water that haven't been thoroughly tested, especially for long term effects.

Environmental toxins used in agriculture also become sequestered in the fatty tissue of animals in our food chain, and in tissue of humans who are exposed to them. Fat from human breast cancer tissue has been found to have almost double the safe amount of chlorinated pesticides like DDT and about ten times as much hexa-chloro-cyclo-hexane, another pesticide.

Even our general drinking water supply is affected.

Carcinogen-containing pesticides and petroleum products leach into tap water supplies from both ground and reservoirs. Even the chlorine chemicals used in water purification bind with organic matter to form cancer causing by-products.

Two of these, tri-halomethanes (THMs) and haloacetic acids (HAAs) damage DNA cells directly exposed to them. THMs are linked to lung, stomach, bladder, esophageal, rectal and breast cancer. (Have your tap water testedif you feel its taste is strange or its quality is bad.) You may be right. Invest in a filter system, and puchase bottled water for drinking.

It's easy to get the idea that anything and everything can cause cancer. Sometimes it seems like we're assaulted from all sides by cancer-causing activators that we can't control. The average person is exposed to over 500 chemicals a day, and this number doesn't even include the person who works in a chemically overloaded environment like a factory. I know people who think they might as well give up, do what they like, and enjoy life, even if life will be shorter.

Is cancer preventable? There are so many factors implicated in cancer onset. We know there is no simple solution to this complex problem.

But naturopaths and holistically-oriented health practitioners believe that since cancer is largely the result of environmental and lifestyle factors, it is therefore preventable. Most of these experts have treated patients successfully for years with a broad spectrum of metabolic therapies to normalize and restore body functions.... therapies that include nutrition enhancement through diet and supplementation, cancer fighting herbal medicines, detoxification, and enzyme therapy.

A person who has not developed cancer can expect that a healthy lifestyle that **inclues a wholesome diet, exercise, a positive attitude** and **toxin avoidance** can prevent up to 90% of cancers.

Cancer is obviously not a single entity with a single cause, but a complex, multi-dimensional disease. Over 200 different diseases are now medically classified as cancer. There is no way that chasing each cancer classification with a drug can even approach the different requirements and ramifications of every one. Unless the environment that supports cancer is changed to an environment that is healthy, then cytotoxic therapies like surgery, chemotherapy and radiation are doomed to failure. They only temporarily reduce tumor burden, and they do not cure cancer.

I feel the only chance for success is to use every part of our lifestyle to normalize tissue that is out of control, especially with living medicines like superfoods and herbs that can biologically address cancer cells. **Keeping the immune system strong is a key.**

How can we remain healthy in a destructive environment? Diet is the first place to look. Dietary factors are undeniably involved with the largest number of cancers, and most experts now believe that proper nutrition can prevent 50% to 90% of all cancers.

Breast, uterine, kidney and colon cancers are closely related to the kind of protein and fat we eat, especially protein and fat from meats, and saturated fats from junk foods and fried foods. Dietary factors are also directly linked to cancer of the rectum, stomach, intestines, mouth, throat, esophagus, pancreas, liver, ovaries, uterus, prostate, thyroid, and bladder. **Improving your diet directly improves your defenses against cancer because it can change the conditions which support tumor growth.** The body has built-in checkpoints to keep itself disease free and running normally, like detoxification, genetic repair, immune stimulation, and isolating and sealing abnormal cell growths. Each of these factors relies heavily on good nutrition.

The latest figures show that nutritional factors account for 60% of women's cancers and 45% of men's. Extrapolating from that number means that good food choices could have helped prevent 390,000 to 725,000 new cancer cases, and between 175,000 to 335,000 cancer deaths in 1995 in the U. S. alone!

Even if your genetics and lifestyle are against you, your diet may still make a tremendous difference in your cancer odds. Whole food nutrition allows the body to use its built-in restorative and repair abilities to re-establish metabolic balance. A healthy diet can intervene in the cancer process at many stages, from its conception, to its growth and spread.

For example, we know that certain body chemicals must be "activated" before they can initiate cancer. Food can block the activation process. Antioxidant foods can snuff out carcinogens, nip free radical cascades in the bud, even repair some cellular damage.

Certain foods accelerate body detoxification, and prevent the genetic ruin of cells, a prelude to cancer. It's one of the reasons I emphasize a detoxification diet as part of a cancer control program. Healthy food chemicals in cells can determine whether a cancer-causing virus or a cancer promoter like excess estrogen will turn tissue cancerous. Even after cells have massed into benign structures that may grow into tumors, food compounds can intervene to stop further growth. Some actually shrink the patches of precancerous cells.

Although far less powerful at later stages, diet can still influence the metastasis or spread of cancer. Wandering cancer cells need the right conditions to attach and grow. Food agents can foster a hostile or a favorable environment. Certain foods also act as anti-carcinogens..... inhibiting tumor development and growth, inhibiting or preventing metastasis of tumors, and helping normalize cancer cells. So even after cancer is diagnosed, the right foods may help prolong your life.

I believe you should consider a good diet as a health insurance policy to prevent cancer. If you already have cancer, you should consider your food as important medicine.

Massive new research is validating what naturopaths have known for decades. The more fruits and vegetables you eat, the less your cancer risk, regardless of the type of cancer. For many cancers, people who eat lots of fruits and vegetables have half the risk of people who eat only a few of them.

Most studies show that even small to moderate amounts of fruits and vegetables make a big difference. Two fruits and three vegetable servings a day show amazing anti-cancer results. Eating fruit twice a day, instead of twice a week, can cut the risk of lung cancer by 75% even in smokers.

One National Cancer Institute spokesman said it is almost mind-boggling, that ordinary fruits and vegetables could be so effective against such a potent carcinogen as cigarette smoke. The evidence is so overwhelming that some researchers are beginning to view fruits and vegetables as powerful preventive drugs that could substantially wipe out the scourge of cancer. What an about-face this has been for cancer study!

Happily, there are almost as many anti-cancer foods as there are cancer promoting agents in our environment. Here is my diet strategy to prevent (and help overcome) cancer:

1) **Get plenty of fruits and vegetables**, especially those rich in vitamin C, for immune support and anti-oxidant protection, like citrus fruits, tomatoes, peppers and broccoli. **Cruciferous vegetables**, like broccoli and cauliflower, are extremely important, because they contain plant chemicals that are able to break down carcinogens and remove them from the body. These same vegetable substances break down excess estrogens that are responsible for some types of breast cancer, and inhibit cancer growth once it is present. **Fiber-rich fruits, veg-**

etables and whole grains absorb excess bile and improve healthy intestinal bacteria to keep immunity strong. Fiber also normally helps flush excess extrogens from the body.

2) Antioxidant foods, like wheat germ, soy products, yellow, orange and green vegetables, green tea, citrus fruits, and olive oil help normalize pre-cancerous cells, and neutralize cancer-causing free radicals.

3) Active culture yogurt helps neutralize carcinogens, and de-activates enzymes that allow body substances to turn into cancer.

4) Folic acid is critical to normal DNA synthesis so healthy cells do not turn cancerous. Get folic acid foods from whole wheat and wheat germ, leafy greens, beets, asparagus, fish, sunflower seeds, and citrus fruits.

Want to get all the advantages of the above list in one meal? Have my ANTI-CANCER SALAD and SALAD DRESSING several times a week:

For the salad: mix 1 cup of mixed chopped red, yellow and green onions, 1 cup chopped steamed broccoli, $\frac{1}{2}$ cup chopped cooked beets, $\frac{1}{2}$ cup of chopped celery, $\frac{1}{2}$ cup shredded carrots, $\frac{1}{4}$ cup of chopped bell peppers, $\frac{1}{4}$ cup chopped calendula flowers (marigolds - easy to grow anywhere), $\frac{1}{2}$ cup of chopped cucumber, $\frac{1}{4}$ cup fresh sage leaves.

For the dressing: Marinate 6 minced garlic cloves in 3 TBS. flaxseed oil. Add 2 sprigs of fresh rosemary, half a squeezed lemon, 2 minced hot peppers, $\frac{1}{4}$ teasp. cumin seed, $\frac{1}{4}$ teasp. thyme leaves. Top with dollops of plain yogurt.

To overcome or reverse cancer, what you don't eat is as important as what you do eat. Be extra careful about the following foods:

** **Fat intake** is the key dietary risk factor linked to cancer. Fat is not a carcinogen itself, but rather stores carcinogenic toxins, like pesticides, air pollutants, industrial chemical residues and the hydrogenated oils in processed foods. Many of these toxins also contain environmental estrogens, compounds that mimic estrogen effects and are associated with breast cancer, low sperm count, undescended testicles and some birth deformities. Testing shows that people who eat high fat diets and are more than 40% above their ideal weight have the highest concentrations of these chemicals in the soft parts of the body, like the breasts, reproductive organs and brain.

** **Red meat** intake is linked to cancer, largely because red meat foods are high in fats. In addition, many food animals are injected with hormones and antibiotics that compete with and block the body's hormone receptor sites, causing imbalances at the basic levels of the body that allow cancer to take hold. (Sadly, although chicken has normally been a healthy, low fat meat, chickens are no longer raised in free-run yards, so chicken, too, is now often injected with hormones and antibiotics.) More than a few women have told me that they can tell when they have eaten hormone-injected meats or dairy foods because their breasts and abdomen swell.

** **Sugar** may have a direct effect on cancer growth. In more than moderate amounts, it causes the body to produce ever-larger amounts of insulin, linked to cancer just like excess estrogens. Cancer tumors are considered "obligate glucose metabolizers" which means they must feed on sugar. Americans consume about 20% of their calories from refined sugar.

** **Smoked, pickled, and nitrite-cured foods** are linked to stomach cancer. Nitrites combine with amino acids in the stomach to produce carcinogenic nitrosamines. Smoking and barbequeing of meats produces mutagens formed from the high temperature burn off. (Raw cultured vegetables like sauerkraut are not considered pickled).

** **Caffeine risk** for cancer is dose-related. Large amounts of coffee (more than 2 cups of strong coffee a day) show significant correlation to cancer, but scientists see this as a factor of the high temperature hydrocarbons used in roasting.

** **Is dietary iron a cause of cancer?** Food products have been fortified with iron for years to reduce iron-deficiency anemia, but new testing suggests that the greater the iron concentration in a person's blood, the greater the risk of cancer. At even 10% above the average level of blood iron, the risk of developing cancer begins to rise. Researchers believe that iron may increase free radical production, a known cause of cancer. In addition, it seems that cancer cells, once developed, may use the excess iron to grow and replicate. Apparently iron builds up over time, and the only way to release it is to bleed. (Ancient healers who used leaches for this purpose may have been on the right track after all.) If your blood iron levels are high, consider donating blood periodically.

How much is too much? The problem is important during pregnancy, when iron is needed to boost blood volume for the fetus, and during lactation for infant brain development. If you are pregnant or lactating, or taking iron for anemia, consider blood work to determine your blood iron.

Macrobiotics have been used in the Orient for centuries as part of the natural healing tradition. Can a macrobiotic diet really help you overcome cancer?

A macrobiotic diet is an effective method of improving body chemistry against cancer. Macro-biotic, (meaning long life), stems from the Oriental philosophy that considers the seasons, climate, traditional culture, and a person's health condition in determining the way to eat. In America, macrobiotics has become popular as a therapeutic diet approach for serious, degenerative illness. It is an effective technique because it works to normalize body chemistry, acts as a detoxifying cleansing regimen, and helps to rebuild healthy blood and cells.

The macrobiotic way of eating is low in fat, non-mucous-forming, and rich in vegetable fiber and protein. It is stimulating to the heart and circulatory system through emphasis on Oriental foods such as miso, green tea, and shiitake mushrooms. It is alkalizing with umeboshi plums and brown rice. It is high in potassium, natural iodine, and other minerals and trace elements through sea vegetables and soy foods.

The most apparent difference between the macrobiotic system and other organic approaches is its reliance on whole grains. It suggests that at least half of the daily food intake be whole grain products, such as brown rice, whole wheat, oats, barley, millet, buckwheat, rye and corn. Other foods in order of their importance in a macrobiotic diet are vegetables, oil, fish, and occasional nuts, fruits and eggs.

Although many macrobiotic followers prefer to avoid all animal foods, macrobiotics is not a vegetarian system and fish is normally included. Other meats, refined grains, sugar and sweeteners (except rice syrup and barley malt in small amounts), most dairy products, infertile eggs, processed foods and beverages containing stimulants, are not part of a strict macrobiotic diet. Vegetables, both raw and cooked, make up 30% of the diet. Beans, sea vegetables and soups comprise 10 to 15%. Fruits and nuts are considered pleasure foods and are eaten only occasionally as desserts or snacks.

A macrobiotic diet's greatest benefit is that it is cleansing and strengthening at the same time. It offers a way of eating that is easily individualized for the environment, the seasons, and the constitution of the person using it.

However, a strict macrobiotic diet used over a long period of time, can be excessively severe for a person living a busy, stressful life in today's polluted environment. In my experience, a better way is to follow a strict macrobiotic diet for three to six months, and then to gradually move to a less stringent macrobiotic diet. A light, modified macrobiotic diet does not follow a set pattern, but rather emphasizes the principles of macrobiotics with the flexibility of individual needs.

One should still avoid refined foods, and foods with additives on a modified macrobiotic diet. Brown rice, other whole grains, and fresh foods, should still be the diet mainstays. Therapeutic foods, such as miso, bancha tea, shiitake and reishi mushrooms, sea plants, soy foods and umeboshi plums should be included regularly.

A note of caution about stringent therapeutic diets:
If you decide to use a strict cleansing/healing way of eating, such as macrobiotics, fruit cleansing, juice fasting, mono diets, etc., use caution if you cannot be in a controlled clinical environment. In my experience, excessively limited diets should be used only as short term programs.

There must be balance to your diet. It is largely "civilization" foods and lack of balance that get us into trouble. A wide range of nutrients is necessary for cell growth, immunity and energy, for healing and strength, for stamina, assimilation and weight maintenance. For the best route to long term health, find out what foods have the elements you need in their natural state, (check out COOKING FOR HEALTHY HEALING by Linda Page for this information) and include them in your diet on a regular basis.

Alternative Therapy Intervention
Beyond diet, how can we cut our risk for cancer?

Can nutritional and lifestyle therapies really prevent cancer or help in its remission?

The link between cancer and lifestyle is undeniable. Every research study points to rallying the immune system as the best protection against cancer. We know that the body possesses some inherent cancer-fighting substances because most cancer patients do not die. We know that certain herbs and other nutritional substances help stimulate our immune response. I feel that encouraging the body's native ability to fight cancer through biological therapies offers the best chance of dealing with the highly polluted, poorly nourished, stressful environment that probably caused the cancer in the first place.

Most cancers respond favorably to alternative medicine methods. Here are my favorite natural cancer fighters:

ENZYME THERAPY

Enzymes are essential in the fight against cancer. In the past, the theory about enzymes as they related to cancer treatment was the link between enzymes and immunity. Enzymes significantly raise the rate of the body's biochemical defense mechanisms to fight disease.

But solid European research over the last twenty years shows that enzyme therapy does more than support the immune system. Successful tests have been done with digestive enzymes against tumor growth and spread, in preventing radon-induced lung cancer in miners, and in reducing the complications of cancer like joint pain and depression. A five year study even showed improvement in breast cancer survival. Bromelain, an enzyme from pineapple, is an inhibitor of leukemia cell growth, and in laboratory cultures has normalized leukemia cells.

Extrapolations from these tests indicate that enzymes:

1) improve immune response by helping the immune system eliminate cancer cells. 2) chemically alter by-products of a tumor to lessen cancer's side effects. 3) change the surface of a tumor to make it more vulnerable to the immune system.

The absence of certain enzymes is one reason why cancer cells are able to grow. Unfortunately, enzyme deficiency happens at such a deep level of the body processes that we don't become aware of it until a serious immune system disorder or chronic disease like cancer has taken hold. Yet most of the time, our body communicates with itself at a subconscious level to keep the healing process going.

Here's how enzyme healing seems to work:

When the body detects cancer, it sends out signals for help. Proteolytic enzymes react to the signals by disintegrating the cancer cells, stripping off the cells' protective fibrin coating, and exposing their antigens to macrophages (immune "eater" cells). They even carry away the toxic debris. Enzymes also diminish the stickiness of cancer cells, preventing metastasis.

The presence of proteolytic enzymes holds cancer cells in check, so **the more cancer cells form in the body, the more enzymes the body needs.** Good enzyme function should be a watchword for cancer prevention. If your diet is heavy in chemical-laced foods, red meat protein, and fatty dairy products, enzymes normally held in reserve to fight disease are pulled out of storage for digestion. Disease-fighting white blood cells where these enzymes are stored are then elevated to an unnaturally high rate and the immune system is weakened. A pattern of chronic fatigue and low blood sugar symptoms sets in. The poorly digested food can block up in the intestines causing constipation and fermentation of the undigested food. Cancer proliferates in this type of environment.

I feel that people with a high risk of cancer can reduce that risk by taking enzymes. Their value is clear, both in terms of an enzyme-rich diet and the use of supplemental enzymes.

Have a fresh green salad every day. Fresh foods are a good source of disease-fighting hydrolytic enzymes. Raw cultured vegetables, like sauerkraut, are also a rich source of these enzymes. Hydrolases speed up the inflammation reduction process, leading to earlier recovery. They also stimulate immune system response. Bromelain, from pineapple, and papain, from papaya are good food sources of hydrolase enzymes.

Here are some enzyme products that impress me:
1) PUREZYME by Transformation Enzyme Corporation (a strong protease formula best used on an empty stomach about 2 hours after eating.)

2) DIGESTZYME by Transformation Enzyme Corporation (use with meals to aid in the complete and efficient digestion of food.)

NOTE: *Any protease formula can cause a burning sensation if you have the following conditions: gastritis, gastric ulcer, duodenal ulcers or esophageal ulcers.* GASTROZYME by Transformation Enzyme may be used until these conditions are relieved, then take the protease products.

3) REZYME by Nature's Secret - A two part program.

Tests with Co-enzyme Q_{10} indicate that it is a key to enzyme therapy against cancer, even in advanced stages.

CoQ_{10} can help in three ways:
1) As an anti-oxidant, it gives the immune system a boost.
2) To help raise body energy levels in cancer patients.
3) In conjunction with vitamin B_6, to help the body avoid some of the damage done by chemotherapy and radiation treatments, especially weakening of the heart muscle

Do you have enough enzymes? The first signs of enzyme deficiency are fatigue, premature aging and weight gain. Most nutrient deficiency problems as we age result not from the lack of the nutrients themselves, but from the body's inability to absorb them. Cancer protecting foods like dark green vegetables, fish, broccoli and soy products are rich sources of Co Q_{10}.

An amazing study at a private clinic in Denmark in 1994 reported that 32 patients with breast cancer were given a mixture of antioxidants (including vitamins C, E, beta-carotene, selenium and 90mg of CoQ_{10}) and fatty acids. After a month, six of the women showed signs of partial remission. The doctors increased the dosage of CoQ_{10} to 390mg and a month later, one woman's tumor disappeared. Even though four of the patients were expected to die, none of them did. None of the patients showed signs of further metastasis and the quality of life improved for all patients.

Here are some of the products I have found successful:
* CO-Q_{10} and CO-Q_{10} PROSOME by Jarrow Formulas
* COENZYME Q10 by Arrowroot Standard Direct
* CO-Q_{10} 100mg by Solaray
* CO-Q_{10} 100mg by Country Life

ENZYME WATCHWORD: Enzyme protection and enzyme therapy are dramatically affected by the use of a microwave because it destroys enzymes. Enzymes are also destroyed by substances like tobacco, alcohol, caffeine, fluorides, chlorine in drinking water, air pollution, chemical additives and many medicines. Enzymes are extremely sensitive to heat. Even low degrees of heat can destroy food enzymes and greatly reduce digestive ability. Heat above 120° F. completely destroys them. Eating fresh foods not only requires much less digestive work from the body, but fresh foods can provide more of their own enzymes to work with yours.

Nearly 80% of the calories consumed by Americans today come from processed foods. There are well over 6,000 synthetic chemicals which are "legally" added to food. And that number doesn't include pesticide and herbicide residues, which appear in the majority of commercial food at measurable levels. It is no wonder that pancreatic disease is common today. **Enzymes are a major pancreatic protector.**

GREEN SUPERFOOD THERAPY

Think green for a healing diet! Green Superfoods are the newest source of essential nutrients for healing from cancer. Even though we're all adding more salads and vegetables to our diets, great concern for the *quality* of produce grown on mineral depleted soils has made green superfoods like chlorella, spirulina, alfalfa, barley and wheat grass popular. They are nutritionally much more potent than regular foods, and in my opinion, they are the best of the food antioxidants for healing. Green superfoods have a synergistic effect when added to almost every healing diet.

Green, and blue-green algae, (phyto-plankton), have been called perfect superfoods. They have abundant, high quality, digestible protein, fiber, chlorophyll, vitamins, minerals and enzymes. They are the most potent source of beta carotene available in the world today, and the richest food sources of vitamin B_{12}. The amino acids in blue green algae are virtually identical to those needed by the human body for protein. Their protein yield is greater than soy beans, corn or beef. They are the only foods sources, other than mother's milk, of GLA, (gamma-linolenic acid), an essential fatty acid. Phytoplankton are used therapeutically to stimulate immune response, improve digestion, detoxify the body, enhance growth and tissue repair, accelerate healing, protect against radiation, help prevent degenerative disease like cancer and promote longer life.

Chlorella contains a higher concentration of chlorophyll than any other known plant. It is a complete protein food, with all the B vitamins, vitamin C and E. The amount of the many minerals is actually high enough to be considered a supplementary amount. The cell wall material of chlorella has a particularly beneficial effect on intestinal and bowel health; detoxifying the colon, stimulating peristaltic activity, and promoting the growth of friendly bacteria. Chlorella is effective in eliminating heavy metals, like lead, mercury and cadmium. Anti-tumor research shows it is an important source of carotenes that strengthen the liver, the body's major detoxifying organ. But its most important benefits come from a molecular combination called Controlled Growth Factor, a unique composition that provides a noticeable increase in sustained immune health.

Spirulina is the original green superfood, an algae that grows in both ocean and alkaline waters. We know that our cells must have protein to heal and normalize. Spirulina is a complete vegetable protein, providing all 21 amino acids and the entire B complex of vitamins, including B_{12}. It is rich in carotenes, minerals, trace minerals and essential fatty acids. Acre for acre, spirulina yields 20 times more protein than soybeans, 40 times more protein than corn, and 400 times more protein than beef. Digestibility is high, stimulating both immediate and long range healing benefits.

Green grasses have the extraordinary ability to transform inanimate elements from soil, water and sunlight into living cells with nutrient energy. They contain all the known mineral and trace mineral elements, a balanced range of vitamins and hundreds of enzymes for digestion. The small molecular proteins in grasses can be absorbed directly into the blood for cell metabolism. They are highly therapeutic from their chlorophyll activity absorbed directly through the cell membranes.

Green grasses are some of the lowest-calorie, most nutrient-rich edibles on the planet, yet some of the most overlooked and underused. Since the cause of most illness is the lack of sufficient nutrients, flooding the tissues with live, organic nourishment from grasses can have a powerful effect on strengthening the body's immune response against disease.

Barley grass has a wide range of concentrated vitamins, minerals, enzymes, proteins and chlorophyllins - eleven times the calcium of cow's milk, five times the iron of spinach, and seven times the amount of vitamin C and bioflavonoids as orange juice. One of its most important contributions to a vegetarian diet is 80mcg of vitamin B_{12} per hundred grams of powdered juice. Research on barley grass shows encouraging results for DNA damage repair and delaying aging. Barley juice powder contains anti-viral properties, and neutralizes heavy metals like mercury. It is an ideal food-source anti-inflammatory for healing gastro-intestinal ulcers, hemorrhoids, and pancreas infections.

Alfalfa is one of the world's richest mineral-source foods, pulling up earth minerals from root depths as great as 130 feet! It is an excellent source for liquid chlorophyll, with a balance of organic chemical and mineral constituents almost identical to human hemoglobin. Today, herbalists use alfalfa to encourage blood-clotting, to treat bladder infections, all colon disorders including colon polyps, anemia, hemorrhaging, diabetes and most recently as an aid in normalizing estrogen production against cancers involved with excess estrogen.

Wheat grass has curative powers for treating cancerous growths and other degenerative diseases when taken as a fresh liquid. **Fifteen pounds of fresh wheatgrass has the nutritional value of 350 pounds of vegetables.** I have seen particular success with wheat grass rectal implants in colon cancer cases. Wheat grass helps cleanse the blood, organs and gastrointestinal tract, and is recommended as a way to stimulate metabolism and enzyme healing activity.

Why is plant chlorophyll so great for people?

The most beneficial element of all the super green foods is chlorophyll, the basic component of the "blood" of plants. Chlorophyll is the pigment that plants use to carry out the process of photosynthesis, absorbing light energy from the sun, and converting it into plant energy. This energy is transferred into our cells and blood when we eat fresh greens. Chlorophyll is in all green plants, but is especially rich in the green and blue-green algae, wheat and barley grass, parsley and alfalfa.

The chlorophyll molecule is remarkably similar to that of human hemoglobin, except that it carries magnesium in its center instead of iron. Eating foods with chorophyll is a powerful way to bring in bio-available magnesium and to build red, oxygen-carrying blood cells. **In essence, eating the green superfoods is almost like giving yourself a little transfusion to help treat illness and enhance immunity.**

Chlorophyll's ability to provide protection from cancer causing carcinogens comes from its ability to help strengthen cells, detoxify the liver and blood, and chemically neutralize pollutants. Chlorophyll helps humans, as it does plants, to resist harm from destructive effects of air pollution, X-rays and radiation, and especially from carbon monoxide in vehicle emissions.

Chlorophyll helps neutralize and remove drug deposits from the body, too. Even the medical community is seeing chlorophyll as a possible means of removing heavy metal buildup. A 1994 U.S. Army study revealed that a chlorophyll-rich diet doubled the lifespan of animals exposed to radiation. Since the days of Agent Orange and Gulf War Syndrome, chlorophyll is even being considered as a protective against some chemical warfare weapons. Powerful endorsement indeed!

Make your own green drink or consider some of these superfood choices:
* PRO-GREENS by NutriCology
* KYO-GREEN by Wakunaga of America Co.
* BEST OF GREEN or GREEN KAMUT by Green Kamut Corp.
* GREEN MAGMA by Green Foods Corp.
* EASY GREENS by Transitions
* VITALITY SUPERGREEN by Body Ecology

NOTE: Green superfood "shakes" can greatly help reverse the weight loss and malnutrition that consumes so many cancer patients who are undergoing chemotherapy or radiation treatment. Mix one tablespoon of a powdered superfood into fresh vegetable juice, or unsweetened fruit juice.

GARLIC
I know.... you've heard it all before. Garlic is great, but it's ho-hum news. Right? There's no question that garlic has a long history as a healing agent. It is a natural antibiotic, anti-viral, anti-fungal and anti-inflammatory herb. The equivalent of **only $1/_2$ clove of garlic per day** can lower cholesterol, reduce harmful blood clots and blood cell "stickiness," protect against plaque formation (plaque blocks blood vessels, causing heart attacks) and lower blood pressure.

You may not know that the newest tests involve garlic and cancer. Tests on environmental estrogens, like those from pesticides that increase breast tumor growth, show that garlic helps the body detoxify the estrogenic substances, preventing them from promoting tumor growth.

Tests by the Sloan Kettering Cancer Center found that garlic extract was successful in blocking the growth of prostate cancer cells.

Cancer researchers at Pennsylvania State University found that garlic greatly inhibited lung and breast cancer in rats who were given a cancer inducing substance. When the garlic extract was combined with selenium, the tests showed almost **a 90% reduction in breast cancer tumors**. For breast cancer, garlic seems to work by reducing the level of prostaglandin E - a substance that promotes breast cancer.

Here are some garlic products I have found effective:
* * KYOLIC AGED GARLIC EXTRACT by Wakunaga of America.
* * KYOLIC FORMULA 105 with Vitamin A, C, E & Selenium by Wakunaga.
* * GARLINASE 4000 by Enzymatic Therapy

GREEN TEA
Green tea is another wonder food, with anti-cancer, anti-oxidant, antimutagenic, radio-protective, antibacterial, antifungal, anticarious, and anti-colesterolemic activity. Even scientists are amazed at the free radical scavenging effects of green tea extracts. Tests at the Medical College of Ohio in Toledo show that EGCG from green tea blocks the production of urokinase, the enzyme that a cancerous tumor uses to destroy the proteins of normal cells surrounding it in order to get the blood supply it needs. A tumor starves without urokinase.

Green tea also protects against the formation and growth of tumors, especially in colon cancer. Topical application of green tea shows anti-tumor effects on skin tumors.

Modern Chinese tests on rectal cancer and lung carcinomas showed tumor reduction for both men and women who drank two or more cups a day. Most notably, green tea seems to be effective against **pancreatic cancer,** one of the most difficult types of cancer to overcome.

Here are some effective green tea products I recommend:
* * GREEN TEA CLEANSER™ by Crystal Star Herbal Nutrition
* * GREEN TEA ANTIOXIDANT by Enzymatic Therapy
* * GREEN TEA bags by Triple Leaf Tea, Inc.

NEW CANCER FIGHTING SUPPLEMENTS

I mentioned briefly the enormous value for cancer treatment that naturopaths are seeing from **CoQ$_{10}$** supplementation. There are four other supplement categories that I believe in for the fight against cancer: **Antioxidants, Shark Cartilage, Modified Citrus Pectin** and **Lactoferrin**.

1) **Antioxidants** - Before we discuss specific antioxidants that help in a program against cancer, I think it is important to see why this category of nutrient has gotten so much favorable attention. It's because antioxidants scavenge (or "quench") free radicals.

So what about free radicals? Are they the cause of cancer?

Free radicals are produced by oxidation, the process by which molecules lose an electron. To restore energetic stability, a free radical has to pair up with another electron. But the process of finding another electron sets off a chain reaction of thousands of other unpaired molecules, that then search for their own free electrons. Oxidation, or "free radical damage" is the result. Just as oxidation causes oils, fats and nuts to go rancid, so free radicals destroy cell membranes, damage artery walls and in the process set up an environment for cancerous growth. Cancer incidence has been solidly traced to free radical damage to DNA.

Antioxidants protect against free radical oxidation damage by searching out the free radicals and neutralizing them before they can damage artery walls or healthy cells. A broad combination of antioxidants provides greater antioxidant protection than any single nutritional antioxidant, no matter how potent. The best program is to get antioxidants from a diet rich in plant foods, and to augment that with antioxidant supplements and herbal antioxidants.

Hardly anybody gets enough antioxidants. We've mentioned carotenoids (like beta-carotene, lutein and lycopene), vitamin C, vitamin E, selenium, and CoQ_{10}. Potent herbal antioxidants include OPCs (Oligomeric Proanthocyanidin Complexes), bioflavonoids generally extracted either from grape seeds or white pine bark (pycnogenol). OPCs from these herbal sources are extremely potent free radical scavengers with tumor inhibiting properties. In fact, OPCs from grape seed scavenge free radicals 50% better than vitamin E, and 20% better than vitamin C. Grape seed extract scavenges free radicals so efficiently, it has lead to speculation that this activity was the primary anti-carcinogen in the world famous "grape cure" against cancer widely used in the early part of this century.

Ginkgo Biloba, currently very popular as a memory stimulating herb, is also a powerful herbal antioxidant. Ginkgo prevents free-radical damage to the nerve's myelin insulation in the brain and to other cells and organs. Studies show ginkgo is up to 10 times more potent in scavenging free radicals than flavonoids commonly found in plant sources, like citrus peels and blueberries.

Here are some antioxidant products you can rely on:
   * GRAPE SEED PHYTOSOME 100 by Enzymatic Therapy
   * Crystal Star ANTIOXIDANT HERBS (with *White Pine, Rosemary, Siberian Ginseng, Ginkgo B., Vitamin C, Echinacea, Pau d'Arco Bk., Red Clover, Licorice, Astragalus, Lemon Peel, Lemon Balm, Garlic, Hawthorn, Bilberry, Spirulina, Capsicum, Ginger.)*
   * GINKGO BILOBA + GRAPE SEED by Jarrow Formulas
   * GREEN TEA ANTIOXIDANT by Enzymatic Therapy
   * ULTIMATE ANTIOXIDANT by Arrowroot Standard Direct
   * QUERCETIN 300 by NutriCology (a bioflavonoid that shows inhibition of cancer cell growth, leukemia blast cell proliferation, and is radioprotective, reducing side effects during radiation therapy).

2) **Shark and bovine cartilage** - Amazingly, two doctors from the orthodox medical world of Harvard and M.I.T. discovered that something in both shark and bovine cartilage tissue was anti-angiogenic. It could slow down the growth of new blood vessels extending from tumors, and block the proliferation of new blood vessels.

It took the alternative healing community to bring the discovery to the people by showing how the active ingredient in cartilage could selectively inhibit cancer tumor angiogenesis while allowing healthy host tissue to grow blood vessels. Since cancer only grows with the generation of new blood vessels, blocking the development of the new blood vessels effectively killed the cancer.

Two products I have used effectively are:
* CAR-T-CELL (non-frozen liquid extract of shark cartilage) by NutriCology.
* BOVINE TRACHEAL CARTILEGE by KAL

3) **Modified citrus pectin (MCP)** - Tests from the Michigan Cancer Foundation and Wayne State University School of Medicine show that modified citrus pectin, a natural food product, inhibits the metastasis of cancer cells. MCP is a special pH-altered form of citrus pectin, in which special extracted sugar molecules attach themselves to possible cancer cells in the blood stream and prevent the cancer cells from attaching to the body's organs. Malignant cancer cells, which spread through the lymphatic system and blood stream have a high content of galectin-3, the protein that cancer cells use to attach themselves to healthy tissue. MCP works through a relationship with galectin-3, to prevent the attachment of the cancer cells. While MCP prevents the binding of several types of cancer cells, breast cancer and prostate cancer tests were most significant, especially if the cancer had already metastasized to the bones.
* Consider MODIFIED CITRUS PECTIN by NutriCology.

4) **Lactoferrin -** part of the cholostrum fluid that comes from the human breast after a baby is born, lactoferrin belongs to a family of chemicals called cytokines in the immune system. Cytokines play a part in protecting us from most infections, cancers and tumors, safeguarding body openings, such as eyes, mouth, nose and other orifices from infectious invasion. Lactoferrin is produced in a healthy body in copious quantities in the vicinity of an infection. It works by binding to iron, an essential mineral used by a wide array of pathogens and tumors for growth and reproduction. When the bacteria or tumor has been effectively starved of the iron, lactoferrin releases the iron back to the body. Lactoferrin molecules are themselves directly toxic to bacteria, yeast and molds.

   * Note: I have also used LAKTOFERRIN™ by NutriCology in 18-month immune-boosting empirical tests as a preventive against seasonal colds and flu, with excellent results. Use 2 to 4 caps daily during high risk seasons.

Are herbal medicines really effective for cancer?

Herbal or phyto-pharmaceuticals, are the oldest recorded medicines and the newest scientific trend for cancer treatment. In fact, some the most exciting news today for cancer treatment is coming from herbal research. Particularly for breast, ovarian and prostate cancer, herbs rich in phyto-hormones (plant hormones) are showing enormous promise for their ability to bind to estrogen receptor sites and inhibit tumor growth, while allowing cell structure to remain normal. Chemotherapy, radiation, tamoxifen and even new European experimental drugs regularly kill surrounding healthy cells as they kill off cancer cells, making it extremely difficult for the body to generate new, healthy tissue. The herbal formulas recommended in this book have a history of success inhibiting malignant cancer growth. Some of the most notable herbs that fight cancer are: *pau d' arco, panax ginseng, green tea, mistletoe, echinacea, astragalus, chaparral, blood root, garlic and reishi, maitake and shiitake mushroom extracts.*

The herbal formula called Essiac has received an enormous amount of attention from the alternative healing world. It is a traditional compound used in a traditional way, but it has has a history of over 75 years of use as a healing tool for people with cancer. **Is it just as effective for modern cancers?**

Essiac was researched and discovered by Rene Caisse, a Canadian public health nurse, who was told by a patient in 1922 that an herbal tea had reversed her breast cancer. Caisse treated thousands of people in Canada who had various forms of terminal cancer with the tea with a reported recovery rate of over 80% for almost 30 years. The herbal formulation (named Essiac... Caisse spelled backwards) seemed to have remarkable powers to cleanse and purify the entire body. There is an amazing story during the 1960's. Dr. Charles Brusch, M.D., one of the most respected physicians in the U.S. and personal doctor to President Kennedy, wrote: "Clinically, after only three months' tests for patients suffering from pathologically proven cancer, Essiac reduces pain and causes a recession in the growth. Patients have gained weight and shown an improvement in their general health. This, and the proof Miss Caisse has to show of the many patients she has benefited in the past 25 years, has convinced the doctors at the Brusch Medical Center that Essiac has merit in the treatment of cancer."

Dr. Brusch further stated in his report that although the active principle for each herb was tested separately, it was the eight herbs working synergistically together, **in combination,** that produced the unique effect and the best results.

Let's take a closer look at the eight herbs:

* **Burdock root** - a powerful cleanser and purifier, improves the elimination of wastes and toxic fluids. It can relieve infections, reduce swellings and can help strengthen the vital organs. It also has antiviral activity.

* **Sheep Sorrel** - relieves inflammation and is very effective in attacking and breaking down tissue masses and other deposits in the body.

* **Slippery Elm** - feeds, soothes and strengthens the mucus membranes of the body. It stimulates growth andrepair and revitalizes the body.

* **Turkish Rhubarb Root** - improves weak digestion and loss of appetite, acting as a stomach stimulant. It helps to normalize bowel movements.

* **Red Clover** - has been used by thirty-three different cultures around the world to treat cancer and degenerative diseases. It contains four known anti-cancer compounds. The main compound is the phyto-estrogen, genistein (also found in soy) one of the most potent anti-oxidants known, with anti-tumor properties that inhibit the vascularization of the cancer.

* **Blessed Thistle** - has an antibiotic effect, with bitter qualities that stimulate and cleanse the digestive organs in particular.

* **Watercress** - is a detoxifier and restorative in chronic conditions. It is a very effective cleanser, toner and strengthener of mucus membranes.

* **Kelp** - is a good blood cleanser, and effective toxin scavenger in the intestinal tract to prevent environmental poisons from entering the blood. The alginate in kelp, helps prevent the absorption of strontium 90, plutonium and cesium (by-products of nuclear power) reducing strontium 90 absorption by as much as 83%. The US Atomic Energy Commission recommends daily kelp tablets to prevent the effects of radiation exposure and its diseases like leukemia, bone cancer and Hodgkin's disease.

Combined in the formula, the herbs supply nutrients necessary for healthy cell regeneration, boosts the immune system, cleans the blood and the liver, decreases pain and acts as a natural sedative which calms the nervous system. It reduces tumerous masses, breaking them down and discharging them from the body.

Today, naturopaths use the 8-herb Essiac formula to strengthen the immune system, reduce the toxic side effects of many drugs, increase energy levels, and diminish inflammation. * The original formula may be obtained from Flora, Inc. Lynden, WA.

In my own experience with Essiac, I found that while it is indeed a good immune booster and all-around system supporter, more is needed for cancer fighting ability in today's world, so full of organo-chlorine chemicals. Substituting fresh American ginseng and pau d' arco for some of the original herbs offered a better effect. Today that formula is Crystal Star CANSSIAC™ (with *Sheep Sorrel, Burdock, Red Clover, American Panax Ginseng, Pau d'Arco, and Turkey Rhubarb Rt.*)

Can exercise and relaxation techniques really help a serious disease like cancer?

Our knowledge about exercise as an immune-enhancer has increased enormously over the last several years. Exercise actually alters body chemistry to favorably control fat retention, a key association for cancer development. And exercise acts as an antioxidant - an important fact since cancer cells are anaerobic (they thrive in low oxygen conditions). I consider exercise a prime nutrient against disease.

Light sun exposure: Over-exposure to ultra-violet rays from the sun can cause skin cancer. Yet our bodies need UV light to synthesize vitamin D. Vitamin D has a long association with breast and prostate cancer protection. (Studies on prostate cancer show decidedly lower cancer rates in southern states, which have more sunlight than in northern states.) Early morning sunlight enhances the healing ability of vitamin D.

Adequate sleep seems like a platitude when considering a disease as serious as cancer, but its importance can't be overstated when you are ill. Sleep is a prime stress inhibitor and immune restorer.

Spiritual nourishment like laughter, hope, optimism, giving of yourself to others, and love really stimulate the body's healing ability.

Guided imagery is part of a science called psycho-neuro-immunology which recognizes that we have a great deal of control over our own wellness and can choose to be healthy. It is an exciting field, bringing together immunologists, psychiatrists, psychologists, endocrinologists and microbiologists recognizing the same thing - the mind's undeniable effect on the immune system's complex network. The body is far more able to cope with factors that cause disease and to heal itself if it is able to manage stress and "hear itself think." Guided imagery is a relaxation technique that helps put the mind and body in an unstressful state. A good practitioner can use guided imagery diagnostically to find out what area of the body is ailing, as well as actively help the patient to envision cure.

Key points to remember as you develop your own lifestyle therapy approach to cancer treatment.

1) **Cancers are opportunistic,** attacking when immune defenses and bloodstream health are low.

2) **Cancers seem to live and grow in the fatty storage depots, unreleased waste and mucous deposits in the body.** Avoid red meats, pork, fried foods, refined carbohydrates, sugars, artificially colored foods, and pesticide sprayed food. These foods clog the system so that the vital organs cannot clean out enough waste to maintain health. They deprive the

body of oxygen use, and provide little or no usable nutrition for building healthy cells and tissue. Avoid commercial antacids. They interfere with enzyme production, and the body's ability to carry off heavy metal toxins.

3) **Cancerous cells seem to crave dead de-mineralized foods.** Starving them out feels like any drug withdrawal. The fight against this isn't easy, but as healthy cells rebuild, the craving subsides.

4) **Most cancers are caused or aggravated by poor diet and nutrition.** Most cancers respond well to diet improvement. Cancer risk increases if you eat refined foods, fatty foods and red meats, and if you don't eat fiber-rich and fresh foods. Nutritional deficiencies accumulate over a long period of time, eventually altering body chemistry. The immune system cannot defend properly when biochemistry is altered. It can't tell its own cells from invading toxic cells, and sometimes attacks everything or nothing in confusion.

5) **Love your liver!** It is the main organ to keep clean and working well. It is a powerful body chemical plant that keeps the immune system going, healthy red blood cells forming, and cleansing oxygen in the bloodstream and tissues.

6) **Overheating therapy has been effective against cancer.** See HEALTHY HEALING by Linda Page, or Paavo Airola's book HOW TO GET WELL for more information on how to use overheating therapy in your home.

7) **There is clear evidence that certain herbal formulas inhibit substances involved in pathogenic cell proliferation**, especially against hormone driven cancers. (See next section on specific cancers.)

8) **Regular exercise is almost a "cancer defense" in itself.** It enhances oxygen use, raises immune response and changes body chemistry to better metabolize fats.

9) **The primary answer to cancer lies in promoting an environment where cancer can't live and where immune response remains effective.** Cancer does not seem to grow

or take hold where oxygen and minerals (particularly potassium) are high in the vital fluids. Avoid X-ray exposure unless it is absolutely necessary. X-rays have a mutagenic effect on cells throughout the body, setting up a prime environment for unhealthy cell growth.

10) **Stress reduction is important.** Relaxation techniques like guided imagery give you a measure of control over your ability to fight off disease.

Alternative Healing Programs For Specific Kinds of Cancer

BREAST CANCER:

Breast cancer is rising at an alarming rate in the U.S. and is now the most commonly occurring cancer among American women. In 1960, the lifetime risk of breast cancer in the U.S. was one in twenty. Now it strikes one in nine American women - about 183,000 per year. Today, 50,000 women die from breast cancer every year. What factors are causing this seemingly sudden, dramatic increase?

While some feel that a partial explanation for the rise is the expanded use of mammography, leading to an increase in the diagnosis of smaller tumors, the fact remains that our sad statistics are dramatically higher than those of breast cancer in all other countries!

In America, breast cancer is escalating at the devastating rate of almost 2 percent each year, developing most often in women between the ages of 40 and 50, although increasingly striking women in their thirties as well.

Diet, hormonal fluctuations and genetics are all involved.

Recently, scientists have added estrogen-containing pesticides, meats and dairy products to the growing list. Unfortunately, these last additions are validating a process that naturopaths and alternative healers have suspected for many years...the assault on female hormone balance from man-made estrogens.

The largest breast cancer increase is in women who were born in the baby boom era after WW II. WWII ushered massive amounts of chemicals and new drugs, like super-strong antibiotics, hormone therapy, and processed foods into American life. The technology for many of these things was developed during the press of wartime, without the normal years of testing for long term health effects. After the war, a great many of these substances were incorporated into agriculture and household products. Most pesticides, household chemicals and common plastics - the major estrogen imitators - did not exist before World War II.

These types of chemicals affect thyroid balance, which is involved in many woman's diseases like fibroids, endometriosis and breast cancer. A far greater number of people have thyroid problems since WW II, a phenomenon that is also a factor in our current weight control problems.

A woman's gland and hormone balance is very delicate. We don't know the long term effects of synthetic hormones on her body. Because of the manner in which the system absorbs hormones, they may work entirely differently in a test tube than in the human body.

Who is really at risk? The answers may surprise you.
1) Almost 90% of women with breast cancer have high levels of circulating estrogen. Signs of high estrogen are:
*onset of menstruation before age 12, *beginning menopause after age 55, *giving birth after age 30 for the first time, or never giving birth, and *having large breasts.

2) Women who have a diet high in meats and dairy products have a higher risk. Food animals injected with hormones add to the environmental estrogens circulating in a woman's body. Vegetarian women, especially those who eat soy foods and sprouts, have lower levels of circulating estrogen and fewer instances of breast cancer because they seem to process estrogen differently....and they are less exposed to hormone-injected animals like beef and pork.

3) Seventy-five percent of all cases occur over the age of 40. Many naturopaths think this is a result of the highly chemicalized food diets that people were eating in the decades after WW II.

4) Being more than 25% above the recommended weight for your age and height increases risk. Fat cells store environmental estrogens, and chemical toxins. Weight gain around age 30 increases the long-term risk of breast cancer, too. A 10-pound increase raises the risk by 23%, a 15-pound increase by 37%, and a 20-pound increase by 52%.

5) A family history of breast cancer is a risk factor for up to 20% of women. A previous diagnosis of endometrial or cervical cancer also increases risk for breast cancer.

6) Women with low melatonin levels seem to be more at risk. Since the pineal gland produces additional amounts of melatonin when breast cancer occurs, a supplement of .1mg at night might be a wise choice if your own melatonin hormone levels are low.

7) Smoking and long secondary smoke exposure.

The newest research indicates two more risk factors:
   ** Tests show that women who work as electricians,

power-line workers or telephone repairers, (those are around electro-magnetic fields), have a 38% greater risk of dying from breast cancer.

** The cancer history of a woman's **father** influences her risk of breast cancer. A National Cancer Institute study found that breast cancer in the father's family doubled a **daughter's** risk. A link was also found between prostate and breast cancers. Risk of breast cancer was four times higher among women whose fathers or other male relatives developed prostate cancer. Certain genes shared by family members are thought to influence the development of both cancers.

Can breast cancer really be inherited?

1993 studies in the Journal of the AMA estimated that anywhere from 6 to 20% of breast cancer risk is due to inherited factors. Researchers pinpointed a gene, BRCA 1, that regularly showed up in families of women who were highly susceptible to breast cancer. Even though the test to determine if a woman had this mutated gene was still years away, the statistics alone were scaring so many women into having prophylactic breast removal, that more detailed studies were done last year.

The new conclusions show that only 2 to 5% of breast cancer has any hereditary involvement. BRCA1 is not a foundation for all types of breast cancer. Most breast cancer is the result of cell changes after birth. Women who do inherit the BRCA 1 gene still have an 85% chance of developing the disease. But if you don't have the gene, you can favorably affect your risk by developing a healthy, preventive lifestyle.

What's the real truth about breast cancer and environmental estrogens?

It appears that there is indeed a clear link, especially for women who live in high agricultural areas like California. Pesticides, like other pollutants, are stored in body fat areas like breast tissue. Some pesticides including PCB's and DDT compromise immune function, overwork the liver and affect the glands and hormones the way too much estrogen does.

One study shows 50 to 60% more dichloro-diphenyl-ethylene (DDE) and PCB's in women who have breast cancer than in those who don't. Tissue quantity of DDT is also higher. Some researchers suggest that the reason today's older women experience high rates of breast cancer may be that these women had greater exposure to DDT before it was banned.

The dramatic rise in breast cancer is also consistent with the accumulation of organo-chlorine residues in the environment.

Israel's recent history offers a case study. Until about 20 years ago, both breast cancer rates and contamination levels of organo-chlorine pesticides in Israel were among the highest in the world. An aggressive phase-out of these pesticides has led to a sharp reduction in contamination levels, followed by a dramatic drop in breast cancer death rates.

Many pesticides, plastics, herbicides and other chemicals contain man-made estrogens. Science is just beginning to realize, although natural practitioners have known for some time, that **man-made estrogens can stack the deck against women by increasing their estrogen levels hundreds of times.** Researchers have long known that high estrogen causes cancer cells to grow. Only in the last five years has anyone realized how common environmental estrogens are in today's world.

What is the truth about breast cancer and synthetic hormones?

In 1995, a study was released announcing news that naturopaths have long suspected, and women feared most..... that using synthetic estrogens for birth control, and for estrogen replacement in menopause and osteoporosis, is clearly linked to increased breast cancer risk.

Even when progesterone was added to the drug, which medical scientists hoped would balance the estrogen, the risk did not improve or the risk of other cancers surfaced.

Worst of all, cancer risk increased not only as a woman aged, but also with the amount of time she had been taking the synthetic hormones. This is devastating news to women who counted on these hormones to prevent osteoporosis. Yet, we know that when the Lord closes a door, he always opens a window somewhere. I believe certain herbs can offer women another choice, both for osteoporosis and for breast cancer, without the increased risk.

Do mammmograms contribute to breast cancer risk?

Medical science bases its current "best chance" protocol for breast cancer on early detection mammograms. A biopsy is normally performed after a spot or lump is detected, to determine severity and treatment.

Surgery in some form is then the usual first choice of the medical world. Even though procedural advances have been made so that a lumpectomy is now an option instead of radical or partial mastectomy, surgery, followed by chemotherapy or radiation is still the protocol of choice. This treatment is usually coupled with a long course of Tamoxifen, an estrogen blocking drug.

I always recommend a second opinion if you have either a positive mammogram, or a breast cancer diagnosis. Test labs are flooded and overworked, often with employees who are not experts. Recent studies have shown that 15 to 30% false positives are not unusual.

Radiation from X-Rays can severely harm breast tissue and cell balance. Although mammograms have improved in the last 20 years both in clarity and reduced dosage, I still hear enough horror stories about swift fibroid onset to recommend that mammograms should not be done without thought or suspected cause. In younger women, the breasts are so dense, a mammogram screening only detects dangerous lesions about 50% of the time. Since even low-dose radiation can cause breast fibroids, mammograms in this age group should only be necessary if there are abnormal findings such as lumps or nipple infections. Even in women over fifty, where the effect of radiation is less, if there is no family breast cancer history or suspected reason for alarm, mammograms should be undertaken with care. **While early detection can mean less radical medical intervention, early detection is not prevention.** A healthy lifestyle should be the primary goal.

What's the truth about current medical treatment and breast cancer?

1) As I said earlier, women thought to be at risk for breast cancer are also getting their doctor's approval for prophylactic breast removal. On top of this, if they no longer wish to have children, some women are also having their ovaries removed at the same time in an effort to prevent ovarian cancer. Many women are not told, possibly because their doctors don't realize, that ovary removal in conjunction with breast surgery can lead to serious hormone-related problems.

2) If you elect to have any form of surgery for breast cancer, consider carefully before agreeing to "convenience surgery," like having your tubes tied or ovaries removed. Doctors often suggest other surgeries while you are "under the knife," in order to save recuperation time and financial cost. Yet, with the best will in the world, many doctors do not realize the hormone balance problems that almost certainly ensue.

3) Many women have very sensitive breast tissue, even to low dose mammograms. Think twice before you have any unnecessary exposure to radiation, especially if you have no family history of breast cancer or any reason for alarm.

Since hormonal drugs are so often prescribed for women today, I think it is useful to remind ourselves what drugs are, how they work in the body, and where their real value lies.

Drugs are part of what I like to call "heroic medicine," because they were developed largely during wartime to arrest death and stave off life threatening infections. Drugs hit the body over the head with a medical hammer in an effort to give it a chance to stabilize, and hopefully start the healing process. But drugs can't nourish or support body functions, or combine with the body to improve body chemistry, or promote cell normalization.

The truth is that we don't know the long range effects of synthetic and environmental hormones on women,... or on men for that matter. Because every person is individual, and because of the way the body absorbs things. Even natural substances work differently in the body than in a test tube.

Tamoxifen, an estrogen blocker, is a good case in point. Since excess estrogen is known to be involved with the vast majority of breast cancer cases, it has been the drug of choice for breast cancer for almost a decade. Yet, we are seeing that over the long term, women who thought they had beaten the cancer, are experiencing recurrence of cancer growth because Tamoxifen does not allow the body to uptake the protein necessary for cell normalization and healing.

Herbal medicines, on the other hand, are slow and steady. They are the definitive therapeutic foods, combining with the body as foods do, and working at the deepest levels of the body.

As therapeutic foods, herbs do nourish, support, balance and rebuild body functions. They are safe when taken in the low doses recommended, and in their whole, naturally-occurring forms. Herbal remedies as foods, do allow protein uptake for long term cell normalization.

We should **respect and use each form of healing in the way it performs best** - drugs for acute emergencies, herbal medicines for chronic and degenerative ailments that require lifestyle involvement, body balance and rebuilding.

Breast cancer is clearly a case where using natural safeguards and support medicines is far more to be desired than surgery. Prevention techniques and immune system enhancement through healthy lifestyle should be the watchwords for breast cancer control.

I believe natural breast cancer prevention methods should be given a chance, especially to women who have a family history of breast cancer, who feel their circulating estrogen is high, or who may be considering the monumental step of having prophylactic breast removal.

The breasts are involved in many more hormone activities of a woman's life than was previously thought. The consequences are enormous in terms of her gland hormone health.

It seems that there is a veritable assault of estrogens from all kinds of sources on women today. The normal variation in estrogen levels does not account for breast cancer instance.

What role does estrogen play in the body?

There are three kinds of naturally-occurring conjugated estrogens:

1) **Estradiol** is the kind formed by the ovaries... the kind that diminishes during menopause and thought to be cancer-allowing.

2) **Estrone,** a conversion of estradiol, also thought to be involved with cancer risk.

When these two kinds are high in the body, there is more incidence of cancer after menopause In fact, **their natural reduction in the body in later life may help protect a woman from breast and other post-menopausal cancers.** A problem with Premarin and other synthetic estrogens has been that these drugs are formed of estradiol and estrone.

Medical scientists are aware of this and add progestin as a balancing factor, as in the drug Provera. Yet even with this addition, breast cancer risk does not decrease, and the risk of uterine cancer increases.

3) The third kind of estrogen, **Estriol,** is the kind that rises in the body during pregnancy, remains in the body after menopause to keep the female system female, and the kind thought to be a cancer and heart disease protector for women after menopause. (It is widely available in Europe by prescription as a breast cancer protective.) It is the kind of estrogen available in plants like soy and certain herbs.

Are you at risk for breast cancer? Does the natural healing world offer any answers? Can breast cancer be prevented by lifestyle decisions?

I have seen for myself that it can. I want to share with you a 16 step lifestyle program I have developed that improves immune response and helps balance body chemistry to reduce the risk of breast cancer.

There are 4 diet principles:
#1)**Reduce fat to 15% or less of the calories in your diet.** Lowering fat intake almost counts as a silver bullet. Especially avoid fats from sugary foods, dairy products and high sugar alcohol. Remember that free radicals are formed when fat molecules react with oxygen, so reducing the fat in your diet not only reduces excess estrogen stores, it also reduces the risk of free radical damage, and allows more antioxidant enzyme response (like from Co-Q10.)

#2)Increase your fiber and anti-oxidants from fruits, vegetables, whole grains and beans. Especially add vegetables like broccoli, and cauliflower, because these foods contain elements with anti-estrogenic effects.

#3)Reduce the meat in your diet. Women who eat red meat are twice as likely to develop breast cancer as women who eat fish regularly and small amounts of chicken and turkey that are not hormone injected.

#4)Add soy foods to your diet. Soy protein lowers circulating estrogen levels by extending a woman's menstrual cycle. Women in soy-consuming nations have longer cycles and less incidence of breast cancer than American women.

There are 3 herbal recommendations:
#1)Add a natural iodine source to your diet. Hypothyroidism is regularly involved with breast cancer. Thyroid imbalances accompany many womens' problems. Some synthetic estrogens block thyroid activity and increase fluid retention.
        Two TBS. daily of dried sea vegetables are a therapeutic dose. Or use an herb and sea plant combination like Crystal Star IODINE POTASSIUM SOURCE™ (with *kelp, alfalfa, dandelion, dulse, spirulina, barley grass, nettles, borage seed, and watercress*) to balance body iodine and thyroid activity.

#2)Add royal jelly, $1/4$ teasp. daily, especially when combined with Siberian ginseng, is a powerful immune booster.

#3)Most important, consider a phyto-hormone rich herbal compound like Crystal Star's EST-AID™ (with *licorice root, sarsaparilla, black cohosh, burdock, dong quai, damiana, peony, rosemary, raspberry and wild yam*) to help prevent breast cancer. A combination of these herbs has shown amazing results for breast cancer control and prevention.

There are 5 recommended natural supplements:

#1) **Add vitamin C**, up to 5,000mg with bioflavonoids to your daily diet. Vitamin C has antioxidant and anti-infective qualities. Bioflavonoids have estrogen-like balancing activity.

#2) **Add Co-Q10,** 3 to 4 60mg caps daily. CoQ_{10} shows remarkable activity against breast cancer tumor cell growth.

#3) **Add essential fatty acids,** like evening primrose oil, 1000mg daily, or flax seed oil, 3 TBS daily. EFAs convert into prostaglandins, cell messengers instrumental in treating hormone-driven diseases like breast cancer. A diet rich in plant foods not only lowers fats (therefore excess estrogen levels), but also helps normalize diseased cells.

#4) **Consider melatonin.** Women with low melatonin hormone levels are at high risk for breast cancer. If you have low melatonin, a preventive dose is .1-.3mg, best taken at night.

#5) **Add PCO's, 50mg twice daily as prime antioxidants.** Here's how PCOs work for breast cancer protection: *PCOs trap hydroxyl free radicals. *PCOs inhibit free radical production by inhibiting xanthine oxidase. *PCOs trap lipid peroxides and delay the onset of fat oxidation. *PCOs chelate free iron molecules preventing iron-induced oxidation. *PCOs inhibit enzymes that degrade breast connective tissue.

There are 3 bodywork steps:

#1) **Regular exercise is a key to breast cancer prevention**, because exercise alters body chemistry to control fat retention. Exercise in early morning sunlight is the best choice.

#2) **Conduct a breast self-exam once a month**.

#3) **Reduce the stress in your life.** Relax more often.

And there are important watchwords:
Limit exposure to man-made estrogens. Avoid meats like beef and pork regularly injected with synthetic hormones, and fatty dairy foods. Try to avoid pesticides and herbicides.

Reconsider birth control pills and HRT drugs composed primarily of estradiol and estrone - cancer-facilitating forms of estrogen. In addition, HRT can be a lifetime drug. It can destroy Vitamin E in the body increasing risk of endometrial or breast cancer, heart and other diseases HRT is not recommended if you have high blood pressure, fibrids, high cholesterol, chronic migraines or endometriosis.Avoid it if you have a history of breast or uterine cancer, thrombosis, gallbladder or liver disease.

Do natural therapies help if you already have breast cancer?
Many women have successfully undertaken a comprehensive natural healing program for breast cancer ... both as an alternative, or as an adjunct to traditional medical treatment.

First, let's look at the breast cancer alert symptoms. See your doctor if any of the following symptoms are present.
* Discharge from the nipples, or scaly skin patches around nipples.
* Lumps or thickening of the breast or change in color or texture.
* Any breast changes unrelated to the menstrual cycle.
* Persistent enlargement of armpit lymph nodes.
* Chronic swelling and sores around mouth, gums or jaw.
* Hypothyroidism, especially in menopause years is often involved when breast cancer occurs - especially if linked to iodine deficiency.

Here is a **16 point lifestyle program that has been used successfully by women with breast cancer for almost a decade.**

There are 4 diet principles:
#1) **Reduce the fat in your diet to 15% or less** of calorie intake, especially fats from sugary foods, dairy products and fortified alcohol.

#2) **Increase your fiber and anti-oxidants** from fruits, vegetables, whole grains and beans, especially vegetables like broccoli and cauliflower, because these vegetables contain elements with estrogen-reducing effects.

#3) **Reduce or eliminate all meats in your diet,** even chicken and turkey, unless you can find an organic supply that has no hormone injections. Fish is fine. Salmon is especially beneficial.

#4) **Add sea vegetables to your diet.** Minerals like copper, zinc, chromium, manganese and magnesium are critical to detoxification pathways in the body. They protect us from the cancer-promoting effects of chemical overload. Minerals are notably deficient in the American diet today. Sea vegetables are a highly absorbable source of plant minerals.

Low thyroid is a regularly involved condition of breast cancer. Sea vegetables are a naturally-occurring iodine source that balances thyroid activity. Two TBS. daily of dried sea vegetables are a therapeutic dose.

We touched on herbal combinations a moment ago in the breast cancer prevention program. They are even more important if you have been diagnosed with breast cancer. Phyto-hormones are plant chemicals remarkably similar to human hormone secretions. They are so similar in fact, that they do not have to be processed to be effective.

They may be used in naturally-occurring amounts, and the body can easily absorb them through a variety of mediums... orally, as extracts, capsules or teas, and topically through a transporting herbal gel.

What are the advantages of herbal phyto-hormones?
* 1. Herbal phyto-hormones are easier to absorb than hormones from foods like soy, and they are so much more efficient. Soy foods, for instance, have to be processed, de-gassed or fermented to be used. You just take herbs as they are.

* 2. Herbal phyto-hormones have no unpleasant side effects of increased appetite, fluid retention or cellulite build up.

* 3. Phyto-hormone herbs are mineral-rich, to stave off osteoporosis.

* 4. Phyto-estrogens from herbs are only a small fraction of the potency of the body's own circulating estrogen. Unlike Man-made estrogens, gentle plant hormones balance the body's estrogen needs, instead of just adding to the estrogen supply.

* 5. Phytohormones are rich in bioflavonoids. Bioflavonoids mimic human estrogen activity, improve tissue integrity and circulatory strength, and increase organ and uterine tone.

* 6. Phyto-hormone herbs have anti-oxidants which boost disease-fighting ability and estriol-rich, cancer-protecting estrogens, which may hold new hope for breast cancer treatment.

I believe women can have a great deal of confidence in a natural choice that is safe, free of side effects and easily available. Phyto-hormones help activate proper homone balance by augmenting or reducing the body's estrogen supply as needed.

Here is how they do it: Plant estrogens are extremely subtle gentle essences. They are $1/_{400th}$ to $1/_{50,000}$ the strength of human estrogen.

Throughout a woman's body, estrogen receptor sites take in hormones from circulating estrogen in the bloodstream. These sites can accept estrogens from several sources - the body's own estrogen, environmental and man-made estrogens, or estrogens from plants. Estrogens compete for the receptor sites in the body. When the receptor sites accept estrogens from plants, instead of other stronger estrogens, it has the net effect of lowering the body's estrogen supply.

Since many women's diseases, like endometriosis, breast and uterine fibroids, and breast cancer are related to too much estrogen, plant estrogens help to reduce the risk of these diseases.

If a woman's body does not have enough circulating estrogen to supply the estrogen receptor sites, the sites can accept some of the plant estrogens to balance her needs.

But how do herbs help prevent breast cancer?

It appears that some of the hormone-containing herbs also have cancer growth inhibiting activity, which allows the cells to remain alive and well, with normal DNA intact. This property is not true of any other procedure or cancer drug available today, including chemotherapy, radiation, or Tamoxifen, the current drug of choice for breast cancer. All of these kill healthy cells right along with the cancer.

Over 200 lab tests of herbal combinations on breast cancer cell lines with phyto-hormone products from Crystal Star Herbal Nutrition show amazing results in terms of estrogen-reducing activity, which helps to reduce breast cancer risk, as well as cancer growth-inhibiting activity.

Which herbs have breast cancer inhibiting effects?
I tested phyto-homone-containing herbs like *black cohosh, dong quai, alfalfa, licorice, ginseng, wild yam and sarsaparilla.* **In every test**, a combination of hormone-containing herbs and other balancing herbs was far more effective in cancer-inhibition than any of the herbs alone, no matter how much hormone or anti-carcinogenic substance they contained.

There are 3 herbal recommendations:
#1)Add Reishi Mushroom/Panax Ginseng extract, 2x daily for 6 months.

#2)Add royal jelly, $^1/_4$ teasp. daily to panax ginseng tea to boost adrenal activity.

#3)Add a phyto-hormone rich herbal compound like Crystal Star EST-AID (with *licorice rt.,sarsaparilla, black cohosh, burdock, dong quai, damiana, peony, rosemary, raspberry and wild yam*) to help inhibit cancer growth.
NOTE: Herbal supplements are also one of the best, most efficient ways to get minerals. Certain minerals are crucial in the working of the chemical detoxification pathways in the body that protect us from cancer-promoting effects of everyday chemical overload. Unfortunately minerals are the most deficient nutrients in the American diet.

There are 6 natural supplement recommendations:
#1)Add vitamin C, up to 10,000mg. with bioflavonoids - as an ascorbic acid flush for the first month. Consult a natural health practitioner for the most effective way to take an ascorbic acid flush with vitamin C.

#2)Add Co-Q$_{10}$, up to 300mg daily, along with Vitamin E emulsion 400IU with selenium 200mcg to relieve soreness and reduce nodule size.

#3)Add shark or bovine cartilage to inhibit formation of blood vessels that feed tumor growth. In a 1995 study on 31 breast cancer patients for whom standard therapy had failed, bovine cartilage was effective for partial or complete response for some 90% of the cancer patients. Over $^1/_3$ showed response with a possible remission. I have worked successfully with CAR-T-CELL (shark) by NutriCology and BOVINE TRACHEAL CARTILAGE by Jarrow Fomulas.

#4)Add MODIFIED CITRUS PECTIN to prevent binding of cancerous cells to healthy cells, along with EVENING PRIMROSE OIL 2000mg daily as a source of critical EFAs to normalize cell connective tissue.

#5)Add L-GLUTAMINE, 1000mg daily to reduce cancerous masses.

#6)If you are undergoing surgery, chemotherapy or radiation treatments for breast cancer, know that these procedures suppress the hormone melatonin in the body, which may raise the instance of breast cancer. Consider a small melatonin supplement of .1 to .3mg at night.

***You may be using folic acid, 400mcg to balance your homocysteine levels. You can also use folic acid to fortify DNA in cells damaged by free radicals.

Exercise is a key bodywork step: Regular exercise fights breast cancer by favorably altering body chemistry to control fat retention which stores excess estrogen, and by boosting fat metabolism which helps flush excess estrogens out.

A continuing warning: Limit exposure to environmental estrogens.

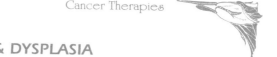

CERVICAL CANCER & DYSPLASIA

Cervical cancer is becoming a common cancer affecting women worldwide. Left untreated, it generally spreads through the lymph nodes to organs in the pelvis. However, nature has put in an "early warning system," for this type of cancer. It is one of the few cancers that has "defined" precancerous stages. Before cancer appears, there are abnormal changes of the cells on the surface of the cervix, referred to as different degrees of dysplasia. Cervical dysplasia is the formation of abnormal tissue in the cervix, generally seen as a precancerous lesion. **Mild dysplasia sometimes returns to normal on its own, especially if positive natural healing steps are taken.** If dysplasia is severe, or in early cancer stages, it can still be successfully addressed with herbal and other treatments.

There are two main types of malignant cervical cancers:

Squamous type, the most common type of cervical cancer, is usually caused by transmission to the cervix through sexual intercourse. HPV, (human papilloma virus), and Herpes Simplex II virus are two viruses involved in cervical cancer thought to be transmitted this way.

Experts estimate that between 40 to 80 percent of the U.S. population is infected with HPV. Long known to be the cause of PID (pelvic inflammatory disease) and venereal warts, it is now considered even more dangerous because it is being detected in cases of severe cervical dysplasia.

Several studies link Herpes Simplex II virus to cervical cancer. A woman with Herpes II is at almost 8 times higher risk for cervical cancer. She also faces the added problem that it can be present and or even advanced in the cervix without her knowledge since the cervix is insensitive to pain.

Adenocarcinoma, the second type, has an unclear etiology. Both sexually active women and those who have never had sex are susceptible.

Who is most at risk for cervical cancer? Women who are overweight and past menopause are most likely to develop cervical cancer, especially if they started menopause early. Women who had early intercourse, especially with multiple sexual partners and a history of frequent abortions are at risk. Women who have taken long courses (five or more years) of oral contraceptives are at risk.

What are the early signs of cervical cancer?

1) A class 4 PAP smear is a clear indicator.

2) Heavy, painful menstrual periods, bleeding between periods, and pain during intercourse indicating the presence of early polyps.

3) Infertility or difficulty in getting pregnant, should indicate testing for cervical dysplasia.

4) Unusual vaginal discharge, often coming from vaginal warts or herpes lesions, raised body temperature indicating infection, and the need to urinate frequently indicating inflammation and swelling in the reproductive area are signs of more severe dysplasia and possible cancer. (These symptoms will advance steadily in pain and severity.)

Women can lower their risk of cervical cancer. Lifestyle therapy should be an integral part of a prevention program. High risk life style factors must be eliminated for invasive lesions to heal and the prevention of more. Even after surgery for dysplasia, recurrence is common without life style changes.

Here is a program that has been used successfully by a number of women, both to reduce their risk of recurrence after surgical treatment, and to prevent further dysplasia.

First: A wealth of studies show that smoking is linked to cervical cancer. Avoid even secondary exposure to tobacco smoke and smoky air pollution if possible. It's almost as insidious as smoking itself.

How should you improve your diet? Optimize your nutrition, especially if you have taken, or are taking, extended courses of anti-biotics, which are commonly given as the medical approach.

1) Decrease dietary fat intake to 20% or less of your calories. Especially avoid animal fats and fatty dairy products. Include soy foods as a source of cancer-preventing phyto-hormones.

2) Increase your intake of fiber-rich fruits and vegetables, especially cruciferous, cancer-protecting vegetables. If cervical dysplasia is severe, a cancer-preventing macrobiotic diet may a good choice for 3 to 6 months.

What foods and eating habits should you avoid?
** Avoid hard and fortified liquors. However, moderate amounts of both white and red wine appear to have anti-carcinogenic activity.

** Limit exposure to synthetic and environmental estrogens. These include high dose birth control pills and estrogen replacement drugs that are composed primarily of estradiol, thought to be cancer-facilitating.

** Avoid meats that are regularly injected with synthetic hormones and anti-biotics, like beef and pork. Make sure the poultry you buy has not been injected.

Can herbal therapy reduce the risk of cervical cancer?
Herbal treatment has been effective both in dealing with the lesions themselves, and in balancing body chemistry to prevent further abnormal tissue formation, especially if you have pre-cancerous dysplasia. Consider adding the following herbal formulas to your cancer prevention program:

1) Apply twice daily as directed Prof. Services wild yam PROGEST CREAM, or Crystal Star's PRO-EST BALANCE™, (an herbal hormone balancing gel containing *aloe vera, grapeseed, wild yam, ginseng, dong quai, damiana, licorice root, black cohosh, burdock, sarsaparilla, raspberry, dandelion, echinacea, red clover, peony and oatstraw*.)

   * Take two cups of BURDOCK TEA along with the gel.

2) Surgery may sometimes be avoided with the use of botanical cervical packs, including herbs like *cranesbill, goldenseal root, raspberry, white oak bark, echinacea and myrrh*. Simply apply powders of these herbs to a tampon and insert at night.

3) Take EVENING PRIMROSE OIL 1000 to 2000mg daily.

4) Take high potency royal jelly, 2 teasp. daily. Panax ginseng and royal jelly together is an even better choice.

5) Take an energy green drink like Crystal Star's ENERGY GREEN™ (with *rice protein, barley sprouts and grass, alfalfa sprouts and lf., bee pollen, Acerola Fruit, Siberian ginseng rt., sarsaparilla rt., dandelion rt & lf., quinoa sprouts, oat sprouts, chlorella, spirulina, dulse, gotu kola, hawthorn bry., licorice rt., apple pectin, and stevia*.)

6) Take the drink with an herbal calcium extract supplement to prevent pre-cancerous lesions from becoming cancerous. Crystal Star has a CALCIUM SOURCE™ (with *watercress, oatstraw, rosemary, dandelion, alfalfa, and pau d' arco*.)

NOTE: Traditional Chinese Pharmaceuticals recommend using the essential oil of rose geranium (*Pelargonium graveolens*), saying that it resulted in a "total therapeutic effect" on over 70% of 135 cases of cervical cancer that they tested.

Other supplements act mainly as protectors. Supplementation should help protect you against the deficiencies caused by smoking, a nutrient poor diet or oral contraceptives. Vitamins and minerals help strengthen against nutrient deficiencies. Antioxidants help strengthen your immunity.

* Take Beta carotene - up to 200,000IU daily. Tests show **a reduced risk** of cervical cancer in women with higher body levels of the carotenes, (alpha, beta carotene, marine carotene, and lycopene, found in tomatoes).

* Increase immune support with anti-oxidants, such as quercetin with bromelain, twice daily, or pycnogenol 50mg twice daily. Other good antioxidents include vitamin C 3000mg with bioflavonoids daily and vitamin E 400IU with selenium twice daily.

* Take folic acid, 800mcg twice daily during treatment, reducing to once daily for prevention. Women with high blood levels of folic acid have lower rates of cervical cancer and dysplasia.

* Vitamin B_6 and B_{12} are protective against cervical cancer.

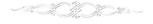

UTERINE (ENDOMETRIAL) CANCER

The term uterine cancer usually refers to cancer of the endometrium. It is diagnosed in almost 50,000 women yearly, and is responsible for over 10,000 deaths a year. It affects two main body parts - the cervix and the endometrium.

Uterine cancer is 98% curable if found early. If localized cervical cancer is not treated, it usually spreads to underlying connective tissue, nearby lymph glands, the uterus endometrium, and the genito-urinary tract.

Knowing the risk factors is a key to stopping uterine cancer early.

1) Post-menopausal women between the ages of 55 and 75, especially those who have never been pregnant, (or conversely, those having had more than five births).

2) Overweight women with high blood pressure are particularly at risk for both cancer of the cervix and uterine lining.

3) Women who take Tamoxifen, an anti-estrogenic drug used to treat breast cancer, may be more at risk for both uterine and liver cancer.

4) Women who have used oral contraceptives for 5 or more years at a time.

5) Women who have a history of sexually transmitted diseases, especially cervical dysplasia or chronic serious vaginal infections like trichomonas.

6) Women who have benign uterine fibroids.

7) Women who are constantly exposed to carcinogenic substances, like heavy metals, asbestos, herbicides and nicotine.

and finally.....
7) Women who take "estrogen only" replacement therapy (ERT) for menopausal symptoms are especially at risk (symptoms are clearly aggravated by excess estrogen). During the 1970s there was a sharp rise in uterine cancer due to escalated use of hormone replacement therapy by women to relieve menopausal symptoms. We are seeing another sharp rise today, as more man-made hormones enter the environment, and even more women take synthetic hormones.

In fact, the most worrisome side effect of estrogen replacement therapy is the risk of cancer. The frequency of all hormone-driven cancers, like breast, endometrial, liver and cervical, seems to increase with long-term ERT.

Three new **independent** studies find that post-menopausal women who had taken synthetic estrogen for more than one year had an increased incidence of endometrial cancer.

The risk of endometrial cancer was more than 10 times greater than in women who did not take synthetic estrogen.

Even when estrogen and progesterone are combined in an effort to balance hormone levels, the cancer risk to the uterus is still 50% greater than that of women who take no synthetic hormones. Although progestin, a synthetic progesterone, can be effective in the prevention of endometrial cancer, natural, balanced plant hormones seem to provide even more protection.

Natural progesterone, such as that found in wild yam, has shown in tests over the last decade to dramatically reduce the risk of endometrial cancer.

This last fact brings me to a realization I have witnessed literally hundreds of times during my career in the natural healing world.

No laboratory can ever completely unravel the beautiful, interlocking complexity of a human being no matter how sophisticated the technique, and no matter how much the substance looks and behaves in a laboratory like the natural one.

When science tries to work with a substance as delicate, fragile and highly individual as a hormone secretion, the job is unfathomable.

I have seen this phenomenon many times as laboratories try to analyze the dozens of constituents and activities of a complex herb, too. Even when partial analyses are made, interaction with a human body cannot be scientifically explained.

What are the serious warning signs for uterine cancer?

1) Chronic, serious vaginal infections such as trichomonas, and exposure to carcinogenic substances, like heavy metals, asbestos, pesticides and nicotine.

2) For younger women, unusual bleeding or discharge between menstrual periods, painful, or heavy periods. Vaginal discharge or bleeding during intercourse may indicate the presence of initial polyps.

3) For post-menopausal women the first symptom is usually blood-stained discharge. Have the uterine lining tested if there is spotting after menopause.

If you have any of these signs, I recommend a PAP smear or uterine lining test (most walk-in clinics do them simply and easily). Then begin a therapeutic regimen to start improving your body chemistry and reduce further invasion of the cancer. (In addition to the program here, refer also to the previous section on cervical cancer and cervical dysplasia.)

Diet recommendations:

1) **Reduce fatty meats, red meats, whole fat dairy products and butter in your diet immediately.** Especially avoid hormone-injected meats. The correlation between these foods and uterine cancer seems undeniable. Decrease total dietary fat to 20% or less of your calories.

2) Add cruciferous vegetables, like broccoli and cauliflower, for their antioxidant, anti-estrogenic effects. Excess estrogen appears to spur the growth of uterine endometrial cancers. Cruciferous vegetables help to manage estrogen, speeding its

removal from the body, and burning it so less is available to feed a cancer. Wheat bran, but not other brans, appears to dramatically lower the levels of circulating estrogen as well. Foods that interfere with metabolism or absorption of estrogen may be partial antidotes to hormone-driven cancers.

3) Eat carrots and artichokes for their protective fiber and anti-carcinogenic nutrients.

4) Include soy foods in your diet three times a week for protein and genistein, a source of cancer-protecting estriol that can manipulate estrogen as well as directly inhibit growth of cancerous cells. Soybean's phyto-estrogens counteract cancer-promoting estrogen much the same way Tamoxifen does.

Herbs and supplements can clearly help:
** **Calcium/magnesium 1000/500mg daily** to prevent pre-cancerous lesions from becoming cancerous. Add *nettles or black cohosh extract* to dissolve existing lesions.

** **Shark cartilage** shows positive results for solid tumors such as those found in uterine endometrial cancers

** **EVENING PRIMROSE OIl** 1000mg daily, with **high potency royal jelly** 2 teasp. daily.

** **Antioxidants** like oceanic carotene 100,000IU, Ester C 5 to 10,000mg, and vitamin E 800IU daily with selenium 200mcg, especially if you are menopausal.

** **A daily green drink for 1 month**, like Crystal Star ENERGY GREEN™, (with *rice, barley grass & sprouts, alfalfa sprouts, bee pollen, acerola cherry, oat & quinoa sprouts, apple pectin, Siberian ginseng, sarsaparilla, spirulina, chlorella, dandelion, dulse, licorice, gotu kola, and apple juice).*

** **A broad spectrum enzyme supplement** that includes pancreatin, trypsin, chromotrypsin, bromelain, papain, amylase, lipase and rutin can attack dangerous properties of cancer cells by unmasking cancer cell antigens and removing the "glue" by which the cells attach to vessel walls and tissues.

** Phyto-hormone-rich herbal combinations are proving very effective for hormone driven cancers. A combination that includes the following herbs is already beginning to show promising results for uterine cancer. It may used as an adjunct to medical treatment. Consider Crystal Star EST-AID™ (with *black cohosh, astragalus, rosemary, licorice root, panax ginseng, ashwagandha, kelp, pau d' arco and burdock root).*
or Transitions PROGEST CREAM for natural progesterone protection.

Lifestyle watchwords:
Stop smoking and avoid secondary smoke. Nicotine secretes toxins into cervical mucous to significantly increase the risk of cervical and endometrial cancer.

Limit exposure to synthetic and environmental estrogens. These include high dose birth control pills and estrogen replacement drugs that are composed primarily of estradiol thought to be cancer-facilitating. Avoid as much as possible hormone-injected meats and pesticide sprays.

NOTE: If you have a Type II PAP smear, take
** A green drink daily
** Crystal Star WOMAN'S BEST FRIEND™ for 3 to 6 months
** NutriCology CAR-T-CELL (non-frozen liquid shark cartilage) or Lane Labs BENE-FIN shark cartilage 6 daily
** Folic acid 800mcg daily.

PROSTATE CANCER

The spotlight is turning to prostate cancer as the American population ages. The most commonly diagnosed cancer in American men, prostate cancer is the fastest rising of all diseases faced by men over 40 today, afflicting one in nine over age seventy. Striking at an ever earlier age, over 200,000 new cases of prostate cancer are detected each year, with the annual death rate approaching 50,000 men. It is the number 2 cause of cancer deaths in men. Serious facts indeed!

Coupled with the fact that male sperm counts have dropped by 50% and prostate cancer has doubled in the last 50 years, it's obvious that more men need more answers to prostate problems.

If you are a man in your 40's or 50's, you're probably giving more than a passing thought to the risk of prostate cancer. Even if you're younger, there's reason to be concerned about hormone-driven male problems. Testicular cancer, which generally affects men under age 35, is on the rise, too. And sperm counts are dropping among younger men even more, relatively speaking, than older men.

Some new studies are focusing on environmental estrogens and other pollutants as they affect male hormones, and put men (as well as women) at risk. A monthly self-exam should be a part of your prevention plan, especially if you are over fifty.

What factors are causing the prostate cancer increase?

Prostate cancer has traditionally been considered a function of age because it is rare before the age of 50, but it occurs in over half the male population over 75. In fact, for years, because tests showed that the older a man was, the more likely cancer cells would be found in his prostate, prostate cancer was considered almost exclusively a disease of **very** elderly men, most of whom died of other causes, because prostate cancer grows so slowly.

However, a recent study by the American Urological Association shows that precancerous prostate lesions now appear in up to 40% in men between the ages of thirty and fifty. These statistics indicate that prostate cancer is more prevalent at a younger age than was previously thought.

I want to clear up any confusion between prostate cancer and BPH, (Benign Prostatic Hyperplaysia), because symptoms of BPH are similar to those of initial prostate cancer.

Hormone changes in men are involved in the start of BPH. As with women, men go through hormonal changes during their 40's that show up in prostate changes.

Just as estrogen production in women begins to fall off in their 4th and 5th decade, men begin to decrease their production of testerosterone around this age. Prostate health is linked to the changes in testosterone production.

Prostate enlargement seems to be linked to an enzyme, 5-alpha reductase, that interacts with testosterone and produces di-hydro-testosterone, a male androgen hormone form **that is also linked to male pattern baldness.**

When testosterone is not converted into this metabolite form, the prostate continues its youthful functions and does not enlarge. However, by age 50, approximately 20% of all men have an enlarged prostate; by 70, it's 50%; and by age 80, it's over 80%.

In BPH, the disease is really the symptoms. The prostate sits beneath the bladder, so when it becomes enlarged, it causes painful pressure on the bladder, restricting the flow of urine. Men who have an enlarged prostate feel the need to urinate often, especially at night. But their urine doesn't flow easily, and the urine stream is weak, so the man never feels his bladder has emptied.

The prostate also surrounds the urethra, a flexible tube that serves as a passage for both urine and semen flow. If the urethra becomes blocked by the swollen prostate, serious urinary problems can result. BPH is uncomfortable, painful and embarrassing, and men feel irritable from the loss of quality sleep if nothing else.

However, **BPH is not cancerous,** and does not usually turn into prostate cancer, even in older men. BPH may sometimes be a cancer precurser in younger men, but testicular cancer is the more common risk.

Is prostate cancer testosterone-driven, too?
Abnormally raised testosterone levels are always involved in prostate cancer, generally as a result of the way testosterone is metabolized.

Men over 40 produce more 5-alpha-reductase enzyme, which converts healthy testosterone into the rogue di-hydro-testosterone. Di-hydro-testosterone stimulates abnormal enlargement of the prostate, but does not have the protective factors of normal testosterone. The abnormal testosterone cells seem to facilitate conversion to malignant cells.

The scientific community sees this conversion of testosterone into di-hydro-testosterone as the major forerunner of prostate cancer.

Which men are most at risk for prostate cancer?
Prostate cancer seems to be linked to certain hereditary factors.

1) Having a father or a brother with the disease doubles your risk. Having two members of your immediate family stricken at an early age raises your risk to 5 times the average.

A 1994 study on men with prostate cancer detected a genetic defect in prostate cancer cells that occurs in almost

95% of the men. The defect, not found in healthy prostate cells, prevents the body from producing glutathione, a substance needed by the liver to detoxify harmful chemicals.

2) African-American men are at higher risk. Black men get prostate cancer at a 40% higher rate than white men. Researchers speculate this is because blacks synthesize less vitamin D, Low levels of vitamin D are associated with prostate cancer.

3) Red meat consumption is a high risk factor. In a recent California analysis of several hundred men who already had prostate cancer, researchers found that men who ate large amounts of red meat and animal fat were 80% more likely to die from their prostate cancer than those who ate meat sparingly.

The men who ate meat five times a week were three times more likely to develop invasive prostate cancer than those who ate meat once a week.

Men who ate large amounts of mayonnaise, creamy salad dressings and butter also increased their invasive cancer risk, leading researchers to feel that saturated fats of all kinds encourage prostate cancer spread.

4) Low vitamin A levels are a risk factor. Enrich your diet with all the carotene foods, especially green leafy vegetables, broccoli, sweet potatoes, carrots and tomatoes.

Does a vasectomy increase your risk of prostate cancer?

As women, we love and appreciate our men for accepting contraceptive responsibility by having a vasectomy. But is a vasectomy harmful? Can you "fool Mother Nature" without adverse consequences?

Women with hysterectomies are only beginning to see the harm that removing delicate glands, or treating fragile hormones with drugs can do.

Science has long debated whether a vasectomy, the contraceptive procedure which severs or seals off the vessel that carries sperm from the testes, increases the risk of prostate cancer. New studies on two large groups of men, **show that, sadly, vasectomies do increase risk of prostate cancer.** In one study of 73,000 men, 300 of the men developed prostate cancer between 1986 and 1990.

The men with vasectomies had a 66% greater risk of prostate cancer than did the men without vasectomies. In another study, vasectomies increased the risk of prostate cancer by 56%.

Here's why: As sperm builds up in the sealed-off vas deferens after a vasectomy, the body re-absorbs the cells. This confuses the immune system, making it less alert to tumor cells. Sometimes the body's immune defenses try to mount a response against its own tissue. In addition, a vasectomy affects hormone secretions in the testes, and lowers prostatic fluid. When the natural movement of sperm and hormones is artificially prevented, a host of male hormone-driven problems result.

What about environmental estrogen effects on men? Are they as harmful for men as they are for women?

We know the estrogen-imitating effects of industrial chemicals endanger women. Men also have estrogen in their bodies. Hormone imbalances threaten their health and fertility, too. Many scientists speculate that environmental hormones are involved. While the dramatic rise in prostate cancer deaths over the last 40 years is a big wake-up call to change our environment, the most alarming statistics about man-made hormones and men relate to sperm count and hormone-driven cancers. While the rate of prostate cancer has doubled since WW II, male sperm counts have declined by half.

The greatest threats come from industrial chemicals such as poly-chlorinated bi-phenols, the PCBs we've heard so much about, as well as dioxin, and pesticides used for agriculture.

There is grim news about estrogenic chemicals and fetuses, too. Male and female hormones must remain in balance in an embryo for sexual organs to develop normally. In early stages, a fetus is capable of developing either set. Hormone balance decides whether the child will be male or female. Exogenous estrogens upset this balance, resulting in children born with stunted sex organs or with a dual set of sex organs.

What is the current medical approach? The medical world has gotten better at diagnosing prostate cancer, largely because of supersensitive blood tests like the Prostate Specific Antigen (PSA) test. In fact, the PSA test is producing an epidemic of prostate radiation and surgery, still the treatment of choice for prostate cancer in America.

What are the consequences of the orthodox approach for a man's life? Radiation and surgery procedures can be as devastating as the disease. Studies indicate that surgery only extends life a few months at best. Almost 2% of men die within 90 days of prostate cancer surgery, and 8% experience severe heart and lung complications.

Both treatments regularly cause incontinence and impotence, because they damage nerves that lead to the penis and rectum. Over 10% of men become impotent after surgery for prostate cancer. More than 12% become incontinent. Radiation treatments frequently initiate a free radical cascade that reduces immune response.

Always get a second opinion if you are diagnosed with prostate cancer. While most elderly men have some prostate cancer cells, most do not die of prostate cancer. It is a localized, non-invasive form of cancer, so life expectancy with surgery and radiation is practically the same as with no treatment.

The European way of "watchful waiting" might be a better choice for avoiding the enormous pain and disability, if surgery is not absolutely necessary.

There is, however, growing concern worldwide about **invasive prostate cancer,** which rapidly engulfs the organ and spreads throughout the body. The incidence of this deadly form of prostate cancer is noticeably increasing among men in their 40's and 50's in all industrialized countries. As a hormone-driven cancer, prostate cancer is especially vulnerable to environmental and chemical pollutants.

What are some early signs you may have prostate cancer?
   * Lumps in the prostate and/or testicles
   * Thickening and fluid retention in the scrotum
   * Persistent, unexplained back pain. (As the cancer out grows the prostate gland, it may eat its way into the bladder, rectum, pelvis and back, causing severe damage.)
   * Symptoms similar to BPH (frequency of urination, difficulty in starting and stopping urination, feelings of urgency or straining, etc.)

Can prostate cancer be prevented by lifestyle decisions?
   A comprehensive lifestyle prevention program that improves immune response and balances body chemistry can clearly help prevent prostate cancer.

Improve your diet immediately.
   1) **Reduce the fat in your diet to 15% or less of calorie intake.** Every study shows that a high protein, high fat diet increases the activity of the 5-alpha-reductase enzyme and thus the harmful di-hydro-testosterone hormone. Lowering fat intake almost counts as a silver bullet against hormone-driven cancers, because a low fat diet causes the liver to excrete the rogue testosterone hormones linked to cancer development.
   Especially avoid fats from sugary foods, dairy foods and fortified alcohol. Add complex carbohydrates instead to fill your "fat holes," like whole grains, fresh vegetables and soy foods.

Vegetarians have far fewer instances of prostate cancer than meat eaters, not only because their foods naturally contain less fat, but also because they seem to process hormones differently, especially estrogens and testosterone.

2) **Limit exposure to meats that are regularly injected with synthetic hormones**, like beef, pork, and fatty dairy foods. Not only is our knowledge limited as to the long term effects in humans of these hormones, but a high meat diet raises 5-alpha-reductase enzyme activity, and therefore di-hydro-testosterone. Foods from hormone-treated animals are exceptionally dangerous, because fat cells tend to store environmental, chemical and food toxins that may be cancer-causing agents for prostate tissue.

3) **Increase your carotene nutrients.** Carotenes from sea plants are an excellent dietary way to get these nutrients, because their naturally-occurring form is concentrated enough for a therapeutic dose. (If you are taking supplemental beta or marine carotene, take up to 100,000IU daily.) There are a wealth of anti-cancer carotene foods: garlic (contain sulfides), red peppers (contain capsaicin), citrus fruits (contain limonene), tomatoes (contain lycopene), broccoli, green peas, celery, and kale (contain lutein) and spinach (contains beta-carotene, vitamin C, vitamin E and folic acid) all cancer fighters. Especially add cancer-fighting cruciferous vegetables like broccoli and cauliflower.

* Add soy foods to your diet. The soybean has at least five proven anti-cancer agents, with anti-estrogenic activity that can retard the development of hormone related cancers such as prostate cancer.

4) Add 4 to 6 grams of fiber to your daily diet from complex carbohydrates, like those in whole grains, vegetables and fresh or dried fruits. **Have a fresh green salad every day.**

Increase your anti-oxidants, such as PCO's to 50mg, 3 times a day, along with a teaspoon of royal jelly in a panax ginseng drink, a prime immune-enhancing compounds.

  * Add vitamin C, up to 10,000mg with bioflavonoids daily. Vitamin C has prime anti-oxidant and anti-infective qualities. Bioflavonoids also have hormone-regulating properties.

  * Add Co-Q$_{10}$ 3 to 4 60mg capsules twice daily, and Evening Primrose oil 1000mg. daily.

  * Add glutathione. It plays a critical role in defending normal cells against carcinogens. It is an important antioxidant amino acid to include in a prostate cancer prevention strategy.

  * Zinc is the most important antioxidant mineral for prostate health. Eat foods rich in zinc, such as shellfish and pumpkin seeds. Take a zinc supplement if you don't think you're getting enough - about 50mg. daily.

Use herbal medicines as primary therapeutics.

The most encouraging news is coming from herbal plant hormones that help to balance the body's testosterone supply.

If you are at risk for prostate cancer, take a phyto-hormone compound like Crystal Star PROX™ (with *saw palmetto, licorice root, gravel root, juniper, parsley root, potency wood, goldenseal, uva ursi, marshmallow, ginger, pygeum africanum, hydrangea, capsicum, and vitamin E*) to help keep testosterone normal, and adrenal and pituitary activity healthy.

  * PANAX GINSENG is a proven plant source of phyto-testosterone. It may help to lower di-hydro-testosterone amounts. I recommend it two ways:

    1) A GINSENG/LICORICE ROOT extract has two potent cancer-fighting components.

    2) A GINSENG/REISHI MUSHROOM extract enhances immune response and has astounding anti-cancer properties. Even relatively small amounts significantly arrest the development of tumors.

Bodywork especially counts for a man.

Regular exercise is a key cancer prevention factor for a man because it favorably alters body chemistry to control fat and toxin retention. Exercise in early morning sunlight is proving to have an excellent therapeutic effect against prostate cancer.

* Consciously take steps to reduce daily stress. Try for more relaxation and enjoyment in your life. A smile can actually boost immunity!

* Go into a conscious "watchful waiting" mode.

Can lifestyle changes and alternative therapies help if you already have prostate cancer?

It appears that they can. Many men today are employing comprehensive natural healing programs... both as an alternative, or as an adjunct to orthodox medical treatment. The vigorous natural treatment included here has been used successfully by men with prostate cancer for almost a decade. Many of these men have been in complete remission for years.

If you have been diagnosed with prostate cancer:

1) Improve your diet immediately. Reduce dietary fats to 15% or less of calorie intake.

2) Add 4 to 6 grams of fiber to your daily diet from complex carbohydrates, like those in whole grains, soy foods, vegetables and fresh or dried fruits. Have a fresh green salad every day. Especially add cancer-fighting, cruciferous vegetables, like broccoli and cauliflower. Add more tomatoes to your diet, and/or take the carotene lycopene in capsule form.

3) Add soy foods to your diet. The soybean has at least five proven anti-cancer agents, with anti-estrogenic activity that can retard the development of hormone related cancers such as prostate cancer.

4) Add a phyto-hormone-rich herbal compound to balance hormone levels. Phytohormones keep testosterone normal and levels regulated. The formula I use from Crystal Star Herbal Nutrition (with *saw palmetto, licorice root, gravel root, juniper, parsley root, potency wood, goldenseal, uva ursi, marshmallow, ginger, pygeum africanum, hydrangea, capsicum, and vitamin E)* has been lab-tested for its cancer-inhibiting effects.

5) Add a GINSENG/LICORICE ROOT extract. Both the ginsenosides of panax ginseng and the triterpenoids of licorice root have the ability to stifle quick-growing cancer cells and in some cases, cause pre-cancerous cells to normalize. This combination also helps to normalize sugar use.

* Ginseng/royal jelly therapy is also helpful. I like Y.S. or Beehive Botanical products with these two ingredients.

6) Studies on PAU D' ARCO / ECHINACEA extracts and una da gato capsules show that these herbs inhibit tumors and certain forms of cancerous tissue like that in prostate cancer.

7) Take CoQ_{10}, up to 300mg daily, and shark cartilage, up to (9) nine 740mg. capsules daily.

8) Take 100mg daily of glutathione, or 500mg daily of N-acetyl-cysteine, a glutathione precurser. Vitamin C and the amino acid Lysine both promote the formation of glutathione in the body, as do substances found in cruciferous vegetables.

9) Omega-3 fatty acids from flax seed or evening primrose oil 1000mg daily suppress growth of prostate cancer cells.

10) Include potent antioxidants like PCOs from grapeseed or white pine, 100mg 2x daily, and vitamin C with bioflavonoids up to 10,000mg daily, zinc 75mg, and vitamin E 400IU with selenium 200mcg daily especially for invasive prostate cancer.

Exercise is a must for men dealing with prostate cancer, as well as early morning sunlight on the body for vitamin D, at least 15 minutes every day possible. (African American men should consider supplementing with 400IU vitamin D daily.)

COLON & COLO-RECTAL CANCER
The best way to deal with it is to prevent it. But America's diet is still loaded with fat and low in fiber, so colon cancer has become the number two cause of cancer death in the United States, killing 150,000 people every year.

Who is at risk for colon cancer?
1) **Overweight men are at the highest risk.** Lack of fiber in a man's diet appears to be the biggest culprit. Fiber is the transport system of the digestive tract, moving food wastes out of the body before they have a chance to form potentially cancer-causing chemicals. A low fat, high fiber diet can dramatically reduce the development of benign polyps that usually lead to colon cancer. **Experts estimate that 90% of colon cancer is avoidable through diet improvement!**

2) **Anyone who eats a high fat diet is at risk.** Fatty meats are the primary culprits. Red meat animals are likely to be injected with the man-made hormones now linked to several kinds of cancers, including colon cancer.

The saturated fats and dense protein from red meats are thought to be involved in 60% of women's colon cancer and 40% of men's. Meat is hard to digest, too, so more of it reaches the large intestine, where it can be harmful. In addition, most red meat is broiled or barbecued today, a process that generates carcinogen-containing hydrocarbons on the meat surfaces.

3) **Smoking, smokeless tobacco and second-hand smoke all raise the risk for colon cancer** (as well as lung cancer).... even if the smoker quits. The risk is dose related, meaning the more you smoke, the higher the risk. There is a direct relationship between the amount of smoking, measured in "pack years," and the development of colon cancer.

A pack year is equivalent to smoking one pack of cigarettes per day for one year. A person who smokes two packs a day accumulates 20 pack years in just one decade! Someone who smokes for more than 35 years is directly at cancer risk. Smokers for 15 to 20 years at any point in their lives are at risk for adenoma colo-rectal tumors, which are cancer precursors.

4) **People with a "toxic" colon**, severe ulcerative colitis or Crohn's disease, mostly caused by chemicalized foods, laced with additives, preservatives, colorants and pesticides.

5) **People with chronic constipation or diarrhea** caused by lifestyle habits like lack of exercise or constant jet lag.

Is colon cancer in your genes?

Scientists assert that there is genetic influence on the development of both colon polyps and colon cancers, because a large number of people who develop them have irregularities in their DNA material. At least three genetic "aberrations" are present in people with colon cancer: one that allows polyps to form, one that allows them to grow, and one that allows them to become cancerous.

If it's in your genes, are you going to get colon cancer?

Not necessarily. Even for people with genetic proclivity, polyps normally become cancerous only if immune defense genes are harmed or destroyed. The body can, and often does, take care of polyp formation before it goes too far. Even when polyps have grown beyond normal immune activity, prevention and intervention steps can inhibit the next stage.

In any case, the risk factor of inherited family proneness is now thought to stem mainly from long standing family diet habits.

What is the current medical approach?

The medical community bases its success or failure against colon cancer on early detection. Early detection can greatly improve the medical prognosis of colon cancer. Most doctors say that early detection reduces mortality 30 to 50% because of new removal techniques.

The current detection tests used are:
* annual digital rectal examination by a physician after age 40,
* tests for blood in the stool, especially after age 50,
* sigmoidoscope inspections on the rectum and lower colon, every three to five years after age 50.

None of these methods detect all cancers or polyps. But, a recent study showed a 90% reduction in developing polyps if they were detected early and removed.

Are the tests reliable? As with every other cancer screening method, I recommend a second, if not a third opinion.

Here's why:

1) Many tumors do not bleed, or show positive results on stool blood tests. False-positive tests for blood in the stool are fairly common.

2) Blood stool tests may show false positives if stool blood is present because of a hemorrhoid or anal fissure.

3) Growths may develop beyond the reach of an examining finger or the sigmoidoscope.

Colon cancer therapy from the medical world is still far in the future even though both blood tests for high risk families and a genetic test to identify aggressive cases of colon cancer, are available.

Fortunately, the natural healing world is "on the case" of colon cancer today with tried and true preventive techniques, and treatments that have stood the test of time for decades if not centuries. Prevention and immune enhancement through a healthy diet and lifestyle, not testing, should be the watchword for colon cancer control.

How does colon cancer get started?

Colon cancer begins as a precancerous polyp growth on the colon wall. The polyp formation process starts with damage to a protector gene. When this gene is deactivated, a tumor suppressor gene becomes damaged and stops acting as a normalizing brake on new cell production. A small pileup of benign cells, a polyp, forms.

Next, an oncogene, a type of gene that gives cells the signal to divide, is damaged. It begins to act like a car accelerator pressed to the floor, and cells start to divide at a rapid rate. The polyp enlarges. Other suppressor genes become damaged, and start stripping cells of their remaining emergency brakes. A small cancerous tumor forms. The last suppressor genes are damaged, and the mass of cells, now devoid of brakes, and driven by the unrelenting impulse to divide, forms an invasive cancer.

What are the early warning signs? You can test for colon cancer yourself. See the self test on page 448 of HEALTHY HEALING by Linda Page.

1) Rectal bleeding not related to anal fissure or hemorrhoids.

2) Blood in the stool, and a change in shape of the stool to a thin, flattened appearance.

3) Chronic diarrhea and/or constipation, especially if there is continuous alternating between the two.

4) Pain and gas in the lower right abdomen, along with unusual weight loss and fatigue.

Can colon cancer be prevented by lifestyle decisions?

Dietary factors are undeniably the largest factor in colon cancer. Improving your diet directly improves your defenses against it

A vegetarian lifestyle reduces the risk of almost every food-related disease, including colon and other types of cancers. In fact, vegetarians have a lower risk for most cancers, because they regularly get more fiber and anti-oxidant nutrients.

Even if you have a family history of colon cancer, and even if you are well into middle age, anti-cancer foods can help prevent small benign growths from becoming large ones. Foods intercede in colon cancer by squashing the rate of proliferation of cancer-prone cells in the intestines, even shrinking small, precancerous polyps. Certain foods act as powerful preventives, almost like chemo-therapeutic drugs against colon cancer.

Maintain low body fat to prevent colon cancer. Reduce fat intake to 20% or less of the calories in your diet. Lowering fat almost counts as a silver bullet against cancer, because a low fat diet allows the body to excrete excess hormones that are increasingly linked to cancer. Particularly avoid fats from sugary foods, dairy products and high sugar alcohol.

Reduce or eliminate your intake of red meats. It also helps to avoid refined, canned and preserved foods that tend to stay in the body too long and add to constipation and bloating.

There are 8 important food watchwords to consider for a colon cancer prevention program:

1) **Make sure you are getting enough fiber.** Fiber-rich foods ward off colon cancer. Studies show that if Americans ate just 13 more grams of food fiber per day, colon cancer rates in the U.S. would drop by more than one-third...... to fewer than 50,000 cases of colo-rectal cancer a year. The best fiber sources are fresh fruits, green and yellow vegetables and whole grains. **Have a green salad every day.**

2) **Add wheat bran to your diet**, especially wheat bran cereal. Even for people who are at high risk with an inherited tendency for polyps, a high fiber, All-Bran cereal can cause pre-malignant growths to shrink. Wheat bran may even act as a protector following cancer surgery to block the return of the cancer, because it seems to inhibit cell changes that stimulate recurrence. Wheat bran is the only known bran that works to squelch cancer-promoting changes in the colon.

3) **Add Omega-3 fish or flax oils.** One of the best ways to stop the growth of precancerous polyps is to add fish or flax oil to your diet. One study shows that Omega-3 oils suppress precancerous colon growth in just two weeks! Fish oils are especially effective for men. Flax oil works well for women.

4) **Eat your vegetables every day.** Eating high fiber vegetables cuts the risk of colon cancer by 40%. If you already have colon polyps, they regularly diminish in both size and severity when you eat several servings of cruciferous vegetables like raw cabbage, broccoli and cauliflower every day.

5) **Eat more soy foods.** Soy foods are available in a wide array of delicious forms today, from burgers to soy bacon bits. Soy foods protect against colon cancer because they contain saponins, components that are toxic to several types of cancers, including colon cancer and melanoma. Soy also contains genistein, a substance which decreases blood flow to tumors.

6) **Eat calcium-rich foods**. Calcium foods fight colon cancer, by suppressing rapid cell growth on the inner lining of the colon... a sign of developing cancer.

7) **Eat pectin-rich fruit**s. Pectin can be found in apples, bananas, pears, prunes, apricots and citrus fruits. Sugar-free marmalade is a surprisingly good source.

8) **Limit your alcohol consumption to no more than 2 drinks a day.** Even though new research on wines, particularly red wines, indicates that they have potent phenols which work as anticarcinogens against cancer, moderation is still the key. More is not better with alcohol, even wine.

9) **Give youself a pesticide break.** Buy organically-grown, pesticide-free produce whenever possible.

Certain herbs are effective protectors against colon cancer. There are 3 preventive herbal recommendations:

1)   Green tea blocks some mutagens, and impedes chemically-induced cancers, inhibiting the ability of tumor cells to synthesize DNA. Drink green tea or take a green tea herbal compound like Crystal Star GREEN TEA CLEANSER™ (with *bancha, kukicha twig, burdock, gotu kola, fo-ti, hawthorn, orange, and cinnamon*) that cleanses the body as it fights harmful toxins.

2)   Add anti-oxidants from sea plants, green grasses, garlic and rosemary. Sea plants are one of the best dietary ways to get anti-oxidant nutrients, because their naturally-occurring form is often concentrated enough for a therapeutic dose.

Garlic is an especially important antioxidant to reduce colon cancer risk.

3) Get essential fatty acids from herbs, like *evening primrose oil*, 500mg daily, or *flax seed oil,* effective in reversing precancerous changes in the rectum.

What supplements help prevent colon cancer?
There are 4 preventive supplement recommendations:

1)   Acidophilus, or yogurt made with acidophilus culture, keeps the digestive system balanced and regular.

2) Vitamin C with bioflavonoids, 3 to 5000mg daily and folic acid 800mcg daily.

3) Antioxidants such as beta-carotene 50,000IU, L-carnitine 500mg, and vitamin E 800IU with selenium 200mcg daily.

4) Co Q_{10}, 60mg three times daily.

Other watchwords that help prevent colon cancer.
* Regular exercise is a key to colon cancer prevention, because it alters body chemistry to control fat and toxin retention.

* Avoid "over-medication" in your life. It's easy to take a drug for almost every little ache and pain, but most drugs impact normal body processes (especially elimination functions).

* Avoid X-Rays except when absolutely necessary. Radiation tends to damage normal cells and increase the risk of cancerous polyps forming.

What natural therapies help if you already have colon cancer? How do you cancel out cancer?
Clearly, many people want to take a measure of responsibility for their own health with a comprehensive natural healing program... both as an alternative, or as an adjunct to traditional medical treatment.
However, as with any program for cancer treatment, your commitment must be vigorous, concentrated, and it must make use of a dynamic army of holistic weapons - diet improvement, supplements, herbal therapy, bodywork and stress reduction techniques should all be used.

Make the first changes in your diet:
1) **Colon cancer is the most diet-driven of all cancers.**
Pack your diet with nutrients. Eat a green salad every day.

2) **Fat has to go.** Immediately reduce the fat in your diet to 20% or less of calorie intake.

3) **Fiber is critical for colon cancer.** Add 4 to 6 grams of fiber to your daily diet from foods like whole grains, peas and beans, fresh vegetables and fresh or dried fruits.

4) **Soy foods are even more important** than in the prevention diet, because they contain genistein, a substance which decreases blood nourishment to the tumors.

5) **Cruciferous vegetables** such as broccoli and cauliflower, and other green and orange vegetables for carotenes.

6) **Sulphur-containing vegetables**, such as garlic and onions. Extensive studies show that garlic reduces developing cancerous polyps, sometimes by as much as 75%!

7) **If you are a man**, especially add fresh vegetables, beans, dried fruits, nuts, seeds and sea foods to your diet.
If you are a woman, especially add wheat bran and beta-carotene rich foods such as those from sea foods, sea vegetables and soy foods.

What supplements fight colon cancer? There are 6 natural supplement recommendations:

1) **With all their media attention, do shark and bovine cartilage really work?** Shark cartilage shows positive response inhibiting tumors from forming new blood vessels for nourishment. Tumors may even shrink from lack of nutrients as the blood vessels shrivel. Take up to nine 740mg capsules daily. Shark cartilage is also rich in calcium, a specific preventive for colon cancer. Nine capsules of shark cartilage provide 14 times the recommended daily allowance of calcium.

Bovine tracheal cartilage helps the immune system resist abnormal growth of cancer cells by activating lymphocytes that slow down cell multiplication.

2) **Vitamin C with bioflavonoids**, 5 to 10,000mg daily. Include marine carotene from sea plants, and vitamin E with selenium and a green drink like Green Foods GREEN MAGMA.
    For precancerous polyps: take vitamin C with bioflavonoids 5000mg daily. Low vitamin C intake shows almost a two-fold increase in risk for polyp development.

3) **A GLA source** like evening primrose oil 2000mg daily.

4) **Take CoQ$_{10}$, 60mg five times daily**, or Nutricology MODIFIED CITRUS PECTIN as directed.

The most encouraging natural treatment for colon cancer is coming from the herb world. Ginseng-based adaptogen combinations are proving to speed healing and normalize cell structure. Ginseng compounds also provide protection from the deleterious effects of radiation treatments.
    Recovery results from people who have had polyps surgically removed, show that they recover faster and build more healthy new cells when they drink a ginseng tea compound during the months of healing.
    Three specific compounds are good choices:
    Crystal Star's GINSENG 6 SUPER TEA™ (with *prince ginseng, kirin ginseng, American ginseng, suma, Siberian ginseng, tienchi, pau d' arco, echinacea, reishi mushroom, astragalus, St. John's wort, ma huang, and fennel seed*).
    or
    Crystal Star's GINSENG/REISHI MUSHROOM EXTRACT or PAU D' ARCO/GINSENG EXTRACT, both of which have shown positive clinical results against colon cancer cells.

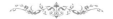

Normalizing After Chemotherapy or Radiation

Chemotherapy and radiation treatments are widely used by the medical community for several types, stages and degrees of cancerous cell growth. While some partial successes have been proven, the after effects are often worse than the disease in terms of healthy cell damage, body imbalance, and reduced immunity. Many doctors and therapists recognize these drawbacks, but under current government and insurance restrictions, neither they nor their patients have alternatives.

Only surgery, chemotherapy, radiation and a few extremely strong drugs have been approved by the FDA in the United States for malignant disease. The costs for these treatments are beyond the financial range of most people, who along with physicians and hospitals, must rely on their health insurance to pay these expenses. Medical insurance will not reimburse doctors or hospitals if they use other healing methods. Thus, exorbitant major medical costs and special interest regulation have bound medical professionals, hospitals, and insurance companies in a vicious circle where literally no alternative measure may be used for controlling cancerous growth. Everyone, including the patient, is caught in a political and bureaucratic web, where it all comes down to money instead of health.

New testing and research is also unusually expensive, and lags for lack of funding. Even when a valid treatment is substantiated, there is no reasonable certainty that government (and therefore health insurance) approval can be achieved through the maze of red tape and political lobbies. This is doubly unfortunate, since there is much research and many alternative therapies widely practiced in Europe and other countries to which Americans are still denied access.

Nutritional counselors, holistic practitioners, and therapists involved in natural healing have done a great deal toward minimizing the damage, and rebuilding the body after chemotherapy and radiation. The program in this book has had notable success, and may be used with confidence by those recovering both from cancer and its current medical treatment.

Antioxidants are critically important to help protect against the damaging effects of chemotherapy and radiation, because both of these treatments expose healthy cells to free-radical damage. **In fact, antioxidants can often help spare normal tissues <u>during</u> these treatments.**

The newest studies show that antioxidants enhance the tumor kill of chemotherapy and radiation **while protecting the host from harm.** (The studies especially showed that natural vitamin E from wheat germ or soy protected the heart against the chemotherapy drug, adriamycin while allowing the drug to continue its anti-cancer activity.) The same study showed that vitamins C and K reduced organ damage from six different chemotherapy drugs while also augmenting the tumor kill. Vitamin C injection prior to radiation therapy provided the host protection without affecting the tumor kill.

Patients who start antioxidant therapy earliest are most likely to live longer or experience remission.

Here's the program: For three months after chemotherapy or radiation, take the following daily:

1) One packet Barley Green granules, or 1 TB. in hot water of Crystal Star SYSTEMS STRENGTH drink (with *miso, soy protein, cranberry, nutritional yeast, barley sprouts and grass, alfalfa sprouts, dandelion, borage sd., yellow dock rt., quinoa and oat sprouts, licorice rt., pau d'arco , bilberry, parsely, watercress, horsetail, nettles, raspberry, fennel, Siberian ginseng, schizandra, rosemary, dulse, wakame, kombu and sea palm).*

2) **Co Q$_{10}$** 4 60mg daily; or germanium 150mg, (or dissolve 1gm. germanium pdr. in 1qt. water - take 3 TBS. daily)

3) Ascorbate Vitamin C crystals w/ bioflavonoids, $^1/_4$ teasp. in liquid every hour = 5-10,000mg, daily.

4) **Co-enzymate B complex** sublingual, 1 tablet 3x daily for hair regrowth.

5) **Hawthorn extract** - One half dropperful under the tongue 2x daily as a circulatory tonic.

6) **An herbal liver support** and strength formula, like Crystal Star LIV-ALIVE™ caps (with *Oregon grape, wild yam, dandelion, beet, milk thistle sd., ginkgo biloba, yellow dock rt., gotu kola, licorice rt., ginger, wild cherry, and barberry.*)

7) **REISHI/GINSENG extract** 2x daily, or a strong ginseng restorative tea 2x daily, like Crystal Star GINSENG SIX SUPER™ tea (with *Prince ginseng, Kirin ginseng, suma, echinacea rt., pau d'arco, astragalus, St. John's wort, ashwagandha, aralia racemosa, Chinese ginseng, reishi mushrooms, Siberian ginseng, tienchi rt., fennel, ginger.*)

8) **800mcg folic acid** daily if MTX (methotrexate) has been used in your treatment. Ask your doctor.

9) **An herbal anti-inflammatory** if there is swelling/inflammation, 2 to 3 times daily as needed. Consider Crystal Star ANTI-FLAM™ (with *tumeric, St. John's wort, butcher's broom , white willow, and bromelain*).

10) **CELLENERGY** by Trace Minerals Research helps break the cell fatigue cycle by increasing energy within the cell, (especially stimulating elimination of cell toxins and waste.)

NOTE: *Keep your diet about 60% fresh foods for the first month after chemotherapy.

* Exercise with a morning sun walk and some stretches on rising and retiring.

* Practice deep breathing techniques so that you stay optimistic and cheerful. Many people have over-come this "incurable" disease.

Alternative Practitioners For Cancer Treatment

For an extensive listing of doctors & centers & treatments offered, refer to *"Third Opinion - An International Directory To Alternative Therapy Centers For The Treatment And Prevention Of Cancer"* by John M. Fink. 1997.

Daniel Beilin, O.M.D., L.Ac., 9057 Soquel Drive A-B, Aptos, CA 95003, (408) 685-1125. Provides complementary therapies to standard oncology. Specializes in Sanum therapy (correcting inner ecology), utilizes darkfield microscopy, computerized thermography, Enzyme therapy, diet, polypeptides, alkalinization, Chinese herbs, more.

Stanislaw Burzynski, M.D., 12000 Richmond Ave., Suite 260, Houston, TX 77082, (281) 597-011. Antineoplaston therapy alters the genetic control of cell function and division and causes cancer cells to normalize or die. An effective non-toxic cancer treatment.

Advanced Medical Group, 5862 Cromo Drive, Suite 147, El Paso, TX 79912, (915) 581-2273. Treatments include: Chelation therapy, ozone therapy, physical therapy, live cell therapy electrotherapy; colon hydrotherapy, magnetic field therapy, enzyme & nutritional therapy, microwave stimultor, shark cartilage, & laetrile.

American Metabolic Institute, 555 Saturn Blvd., Building B, M/S 432, San Diego, CA 92154, (800) 388-1083. Treatments include: Nutrition program, detoxification program, digestive enzymes, herbs, homeopathy, colonics, bioelectrical medicine, ultrasound, ozone, chelation, magnetic therapy & immunology.

Carolina Center for Bio-Oxidative Medicine, 4505 Fair Meadow Lane, Suite 111, Raleigh, NC 27607, (800) 473-9812. Treatments include: Ozone, IV (EDTA chelation, Vit. C, H_2O_2, minerals), diet, herbal detoxification, hydrotherapy, lab testing & digestive analysis.

Center for Progressive Medicine, Pinnacle Place, Suite 210, 10 McKown Rd., Albany, NY 12203, (518) 435-0082. Chelation therapy, dietary modification, herbal & Chinese remedies, enzyme potentiated desensitization, homeopathic medicine, photooxidation, more.

Environmental and Preventive Health Center of Atlanta, 3833 Roswell Rd., Suite 110, Atlanta, GA 30342, (404) 841-0088. Stephen b. Edelson, M.D. Treatments include: Preventive nutrition, ultraviolet blood irradiation, intravenous hydrogen peroxide, Vit. C, amygdalin (laetrile), shark cartilage, coffee enemas and other nontoxic treatments.

Genesis West Research Institute for Biological Medicine, P.O. Box 3460, Chula Vista, CA 91909-0004, (619) 424-9552. Treatments include: Ozone, ultraviolet blood irradiation, Rife frequency, immunotherapy, IV's, enzyme & metabolic therapies, colon restoration, amino acid/electrolyte & HCL pH balancing & hyperthermia.

Gerson Healing Centers of America, P.O. Box 430, Bonita, CA 91902, (619) 585-7600. Treatments include: Full Gerson therapy. All foods are from organic vegetables & fruits, freshly prepared juices, intensive detoxification, coffee enemas, minerals, enzymes, liver extract, B12, botanicals, acupuncture, chiropractic, massage, & others.

Hospital Santa Monica, 880 Canarios Court, Suite 210, Chula Vista, CA 91910, (800) 359-6547. Founded by Kurt W. Donsbach, D.C., N.D., Ph.D. Treatments include: Ozone & hydrogen peroxide, photoluminescence, nutritional therapy, bovine cartilage, hyperthermia, biomagnetics, colonics, IV chelation, and modified citrus pectin.

Mantell Medical Clinic, 6505 Mars Rd. Cranberry Township, PA 16066-5109, (412) 776-5610. Donald Mantell, M.D. Treatments include: Multifaceted metabolic approach, diet, vitamins, minerals, enzymes, herbs, homeopathy, IV (DMSO and Vit. C), colonic irrigation, electro-acupuncture, chelation, clinical ecology & neural therapy (for pain).

Preventive Medical Center of Marin, Inc. 25 Mitchell Boulevard, Suite 8, San Rafael, CA 94903. (415) 472-2343 Elson M. Haas, M.D. Treatments include: Multidisciplinary programs, wide range of nutritional & herbal therapies, detoxification practices, osteopathy & manipulation, acupuncture & Chinese herbal therapy, bodywork & psychotherapy.

International Medical Center (Mex.) contact: 1501 Arizona St. 1-E, El Paso, TX 79902, (800) 621-8924. Treatments include: Chelation, hyperbaric oxygen, ozone, enzyme & nutritional therapy, immunotherapy, detox, electrotherapy, colon therapy, cartilage, acupuncture.